PAIN-FREE PERIODS

PAIN-FREE PERIODS:

Banish Menstrual Misery, Fight Fibroids, and Get Your Life Back

SUZANNE SLONIM, MD

painfreeperiodsnow.com

Disclaimer and Copyright Information

This book is not to be considered a replacement for medical advice, diagnosis, or treatment, nor is it intended to treat, cure, or address any specific diseases or medical conditions. The information contained herein is intended to be for informational purposes only, and any readers of the material choose to implement the information into their lifestyles at their own risk. We strongly recommend consultation with your doctor or primary care physician before making any lifestyle changes. Please always use your best judgment and seek the advice of your health professionals as needed.

By reading this guide, you expressly acknowledge and agree that neither the author, Suzanne Slonim, MD nor the author's company, Suzanne Slonim Enterprises, LLC is responsible for any express or implied results or guarantees relating to any information presented in the guide. Furthermore, any statements or claims about the possible health benefits conferred by any supplements, medications or procedures are not intended to diagnose, treat, cure, or prevent any disease, medical condition, or injury.

Most of the outbound links here and on Dr. Slonim's website are purely for informational purposes. However, Suzanne Slonim Enterprises, LLC may earn a commission on some of the resources provided herein and on any websites owned, listed, or promoted by Suzanne Slonim Enterprises, LLC. As always, neither Suzanne Slonim, MD nor Suzanne Slonim Enterprises, LLC will generally recommend a resource Suzanne Slonim, MD cannot personally vouch for. However, neither Suzanne Slonim Enterprises, LLC nor its author, Suzanne Slonim, MD provide any guarantees or warranties relating to the accuracy, effectiveness, or trustworthiness of any recommended products or resources.

Names of patients whose stories were included in this book as examples have been changed to protect their privacy.

Copyright 2018 Suzanne Slonim Enterprises, LLC. All rights reserved.

ISBN: 978-1-7329445-2-7

Library of Congress Control Number: 2018912896

CONTENTS

ACKNOWLEDGMENTS

I'd like to thank everyone who made it possible for this book to be written. Drs. Ralph and Roberta Slonim have been my life-long role models and inspiration. I can never thank them enough. Pam Gerber's support provides me with the energy that keeps me going. She makes everything in my life better. Dr. Kelli Beingesser is my rock. And so are Dr. Sheba Meymandi and Dr. Shaun Samuels. But mostly Kelli. Lea Ellermeier is my writing role model and a great friend. Dr. Mike Dake is my mentor and taught me I can do anything in IR. Sylvie McCracken is my writing coach extraordinaire. Drs. Danny Chan and Jaryd Stein gave me my start in this fibroid practice. Kimberly Wallace-Gutierrez was instrumental in growing the fibroid practice from the beginning. Dr. Kate O'Hanlan shared some surgical secrets that really elevated my patients' experience. Dr. Gail Newel and Dr. Sheila Chhutani helped me with editing and adding the perspective of gynecologists. Gail Warrior opened her heart and her network to help spread the word about treating fibroids without surgery. Corey Cleghorn's innovative marketing helped spread the word to a broader audience. Anna Butler, Debra Peak-Haynes, and Carina Gonzalez have been true ambassadors. Eloy Zamora makes my work life more enjoyable and fun. Dr. Joseph Carlos was the first gynecologist to send a fibroid patient to my new practice. Dr. Quanita Crable has always been there to provide exceptionally skilled surgical care to my patients who need it. Dr. Hampton Richards is opening all kinds of new doors. Wick Allison is an ongoing source of wisdom. And Knox Burnley is a reminder of what it's all about.

ABOUT THE
AUTHOR

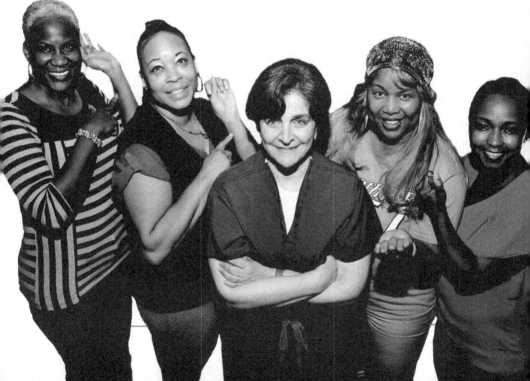

Dr. Slonim with a few of her patients.
They are pointing at the puncture site
for their UFE procedures.

*D*r. Suzanne Slonim was born in Miami and lived in several areas around the country through her ten years of postgraduate medical training. She practices in a field called interventional radiology, treating all types of diseases and medical problems through minimally invasive, image-guided procedures. She received this sub-specialized training at Stanford University Medical Center, where all varieties of cutting-edge procedures are performed.

After several years of teaching these techniques at Stanford, Dr. Slonim settled in Dallas, where she served as Director of Interventional Radiology at Methodist Dallas Medical Center for over 15 years. She was also president of the medical staff.

Dr. Slonim has now transitioned her practice to focusing entirely on treating uterine fibroids. She is passionate about informing women that fibroids can be treated without surgery. She empowers each woman to stop suffering in silence and to make the best-informed decisions for her personal lifestyle and needs.

Dr. Slonim has performed over 30,000 procedures during her career. When she's not working, she enjoys spending time with her family and friends, listening to audio books, watching movies, working out, and watching her backyard chickens.

INTRODUCTION

I want to tell you a real-life success story.

Jasmine, a forty-four-year-old African-American woman, came to see me at my office in Dallas with her daughter in tow. She was at the end of her rope with her periods and wanted to discuss treatment for her uterine fibroids. She had four children and did not plan to get pregnant again. She had a very heavy flow during her menstrual periods, passing clots and requiring a full box of sanitary pads each day. Her periods lasted 14 days. She had become very anemic due to the heavy blood loss and had recently been in the hospital. She had become so weak she had needed a blood transfusion. It wasn't even the first time this had happened; she had also needed a blood transfusion just a few years earlier. At that time, she had been told she had fibroids and needed a hysterectomy.

Those are frightening words for any woman to hear.

Jasmine was worried, not just because she was afraid to have surgery, but because she was unable to take time off work. She was tearful during the visit because she was so sure she would not be able to afford treatment for her fibroids.

The idea of not being treated, however, was just as daunting. In addition to the heavy bleeding, she also had bad cramping pain with her periods, pelvic pressure, and back pain. Her symptoms were getting worse, to the point that she had started needing to wear Depends each day during her cycles.

After evaluating her, we decided that her best treatment option was Uterine Fibroid Embolization (UFE). She was delighted to learn that the procedure could be performed in our office and that she could go home the same day. UFE was covered by her insurance too. She was over the moon. For the first time, she had hope.

After the procedure, Jasmine's symptoms began to improve. At her last follow-up visit four months after the UFE, her menstrual flow was down to five days, she was no longer passing clots, her pelvic pressure and back pain were gone, and her menstrual cramps were much improved. It has now been over two years since her treatment. She hasn't needed another blood transfusion, she's no longer anemic, and she hasn't ever had to wear Depends again. She's very happy with her results.

Women often emerge from adolescence with the age-old notion that menses is a woman's "curse." Your mother may have taught you that women simply have to suffer (just as your grandmother taught her). I'm here to tell you that if you have fibroids like Jasmine, you don't have to put up with your symptoms any longer. There are new procedures, like UFE, that can truly change your life and they are not as costly or complicated as you might think.

If you want to find out how to rid yourself of your symptoms and feel better, read on. Medical science has your back, girl. And I'm here to guide you through your options.

Chapter 1

WHAT'S NORMAL... AND WHAT'S NOT?

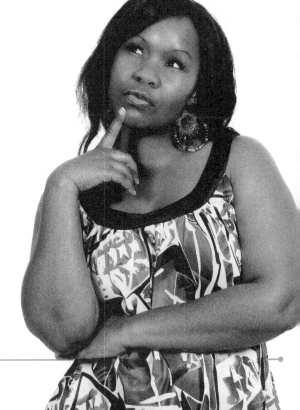

*W*hen it comes to menstrual flow, cramping, and pain, you may be wondering whether the symptoms you have been experiencing are significant in their severity or not. Although all women are a little different in their menstrual patterns, let's go over what is considered "normal" and what is not.

Normal Menstrual Cycles

Most women have menstrual cycles that last between three and seven days, with most of the bleeding occurring within the first three days. The normal amount of time between periods is 22 to 35 days. The average amount of blood a woman loses during her cycle is six to eight teaspoons (30 to 40 ml). Usually there should not be any bleeding or spotting between periods, although rarely, a woman may have a small amount of spotting at the time of ovulation in the middle of her cycle.

Women with menstrual cycles that behave within these ranges usually find that their pain, discomfort, and inconvenience are manageable.

Abnormal Menstrual Cycles

Your bleeding would begin to be considered abnormal if it reaches 16 teaspoons per cycle (80 ml). Only 10% of women bleed more than 16 teaspoons, and of these women, 65% have anemia. A significant proportion of women who bleed less than 12 teaspoons consider their cycles to be heavy, so doctors can have a hard time assessing how accurate a patient's perception is. Most doctors prefer to define "abnormal" menstrual bleeding as excessive menstrual blood loss which interferes with a woman's physical, social, or emotional quality of life. In other words, if your life begins to revolve around managing your period, keeping you from doing what you need and would like to do while it is occurring, that's abnormal.

Pain during menstrual periods is very common. The pain is usually limited to the first two to three days of the cycle. Menstrual pain is most common in young women and it often improves as a woman gets older. Despite the frequency of menstrual pain, it is often neglected by doctors and endured by women, who may come to see it as a normal part of the menstrual cycle. They simply accept it and tough it out.

Why More Women Should Seek Treatment for Abnormal Periods

About 30% of women have abnormally heavy periods, and up to 95% of women have menstrual pain. One in three visits to gynecologists among premenopausal women is for abnormal bleeding and it accounts for over 70% of visits among perimenopausal and postmenopausal women. Up to 55% of women with heavy periods have reported taking time off work, often several days a month around the time of their periods.

The estimated annual medical cost of abnormal bleeding is approximately $1 billion. This amount includes the cost of doctor's visits, medications, and treatments. The indirect cost associated with heavy periods is estimated to be over $12 billion per year.[1]

Having heavy periods is the most common cause of iron deficiency anemia in developed countries like the United States. Anemia can cause weakness, fatigue, lack of concentration, and mood swings. It's a big deal. Multiple studies have shown that heavy menstrual bleeding can cause deterioration of women's quality of life in the areas of physical and emotional wellbeing, productivity, and carrying out daily activities. Women's family life, physical health, work life, psychological health, sex life, and social life have all been shown to suffer.

> About 30% of women have abnormally heavy periods, and up to 95% of women have menstrual pain.

Many women simply suffer through heavy menstrual periods and pain without ever asking their doctor for help. We know from studies in the '80s and '90s that only approximately 25% of women with these symptoms actually seek medical care. We live in an empowering age, however. Now that information is more freely available to women, especially on

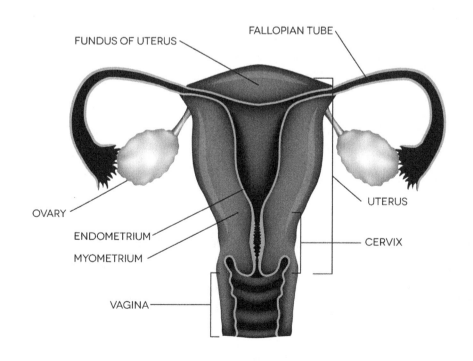

the internet, they have an opportunity to educate themselves and get treatment that their mamas never had.

For about 50% of women with menstrual pain, the cause is simply increased contractility of the uterus associated with the normal hormonal and chemical shifts of the menstrual cycle. That is, when the uterus is signaled to contract to expel blood, those contractions, or cramps, hurt. But when women have an abnormal amount of bleeding with their period, bleeding between periods, pain between periods, pain during sex, or have an abnormal pelvic exam, other causes for the symptoms should be considered.

The possible causes for extraordinary menstrual pain and bleeding include fibroids, polyps, endometriosis, adenomyosis, pelvic varicose veins (pelvic congestion syndrome), ovary malfunction, abnormal blood clotting, cancer, and a few other unusual causes. We are going to explore all of them in the course of this book.

Normal Uterine Anatomy

Before we delve into the possible causes of your abnormal menstrual symptoms, let's review what a normal uterus does and looks like.

The uterus is, of course, the female pelvic organ associated with reproduction—the womb. It is shaped like an inverted triangle and has a muscular wall called the myometrium. There is a thin glandular inner lining called the endometrium and a fibrous outer lining called the parametrium, or serosa. The top of the uterus is called the fundus. The bottom of the uterus is called the cervix, which is a rounded channel that opens to the vagina.

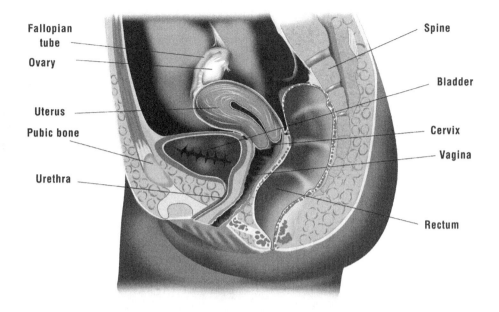

From each of the upper corners of the uterus a tube extends out to the sides to the ovaries. These are the fallopian tubes, through which the egg travels to get into the uterus after the ovary releases it. The uterus sits directly behind the bladder and directly in front of the rectum.

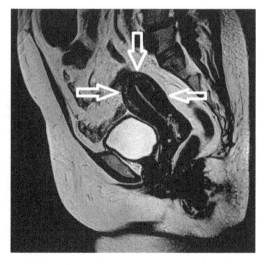

You can use all the images above as a point of reference for what the ideal uterus looks like. If you are having abnormal symptoms, your uterus probably does not look like these textbook versions. But that's okay—that's why we are here.

The arrows point at the uterus.

Chapter 2

WHAT ARE FIBROIDS, AND WHY DO SOME WOMEN GET THEM?

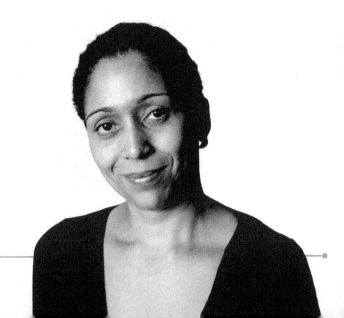

The Basics

Fibroids are the most common benign (i.e., non-cancerous) tumors in premenopausal women. They are also called leiomyomas or myomas. Fibroids consist of muscle cells combined with variable amounts of collagen and other components of fibrous connective tissue, forming a lump within the uterus. Over 80% of black women and 70% of white women develop fibroids by age 50,[2] although only 20–40% of these women will have significant symptoms.

We've been aware of fibroids for a long time. They were first described in the medical literature in the 16th century. The difference between you and these ladies from long ago? Back then, there was very little a woman could do to ease her suffering. You are lucky to live when you do!

The medical community knows there are a lot of complex factors involved in what causes fibroids to form, but the specifics of exactly how it happens have not been worked out. Several different molecules, proteins, growth factors, receptors, and genes have been implicated. As a fibroid grows, it compresses the surrounding tissues of the uterine wall, including normal muscle cells, collagen, and blood vessels. A fibroid will displace the normal tissues of the uterus, but it does not usually interfere with the ability of the uterus to contract. There are receptors on fibroid cells that are influenced by estrogen and progesterone, which explains why these hormones and chemicals similar to them have an effect on the fibroids.

Estrogen and progesterone are essential for fibroids to grow. Estrogen is generally considered to be the most important element in fibroid growth. There is some evidence that progesterone triggers fibroid cells to grow and keeps them from dying on schedule. Estrogen activates cells called fibroblasts that play a key role in over-producing collagen and other components of fibrous tissue.

Other elements involved in causing fibroids include growth factors, chemicals that influence the development of blood vessels to supply the fibroids, and factors that keep fibroid cells from dying at a normal rate. Fibroid cells have a different genetic makeup than normal muscle cells in the uterus. These differences cause them to have higher levels of estrogen and progesterone receptors on their surface than normal cells.

What Are the Risk Factors for Fibroids?

Multiple studies have been conducted into the complex combination of factors that could be involved in causing fibroids.[3-6] Some of the connections science has made here may surprise you.

Race / Ethnicity

There are significant racial and ethnic differences in the occurrence and severity of fibroids. These differences have been attributed to disparities in genetics, socioeconomic status, access to healthcare, and environmental exposures, but the underlying cause is unknown. Possible causes include racial differences in the genetics affecting fibroids and broad cultural differences between the races. Almost all studies comparing features of fibroids in different races have compared white and black women, so there is much less information about other races.

Black women have it the toughest. Statistically, they have more fibroids, bigger fibroids, and more enlargement of their uterus than white women. In black women, fibroids grow faster and cause more symptoms. After pregnancy, when fibroids often shrink, they shrink slower in black women.

Black women develop fibroid symptoms 10 to 15 years earlier than white women. As women get older, fibroids tend to grow slower in white women but not in black women. Black women have higher rates of hospitalization and surgery for fibroids. After fibroid surgery, black women are more likely to have complications and require a blood transfusion.

The available data suggest the rate of fibroids in Hispanic women falls somewhere between whites and blacks, and Asian women are least likely to have them.

Family History

While you can't blame your symptoms on your mom or sis, if a woman's mother or sister has fibroids, she is more likely to have fibroids herself. Women with a family history of fibroids tend to be diagnosed themselves at a younger age and have multiple fibroids. There is a higher risk of both women in a set of twins having fibroids if they are identical twins rather than in fraternal twins. Clearly, genetics plays a role. But the likelihood of

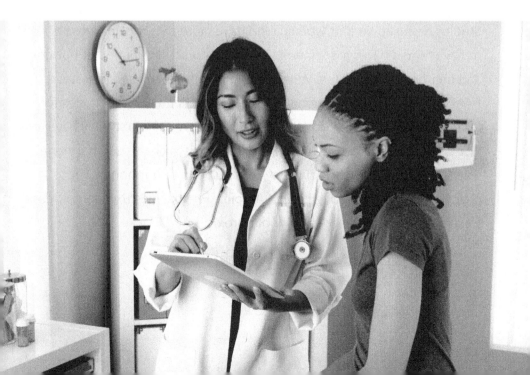

twins having similar cultural experiences and environmental exposures make it difficult to define the relative importance of factors involved in family history.

Age
Fibroids do not occur before puberty. From puberty on, the risk of fibroids increases with age. Although the exact hormonal pathways have not been defined, the development and growth of fibroids are thought to be directly related to estrogen, with progesterone playing a synergistic role. The longer a woman is exposed to estrogen, the higher the risk of fibroids.

Age of First Menstrual Period
Several studies have shown that women who started having periods at an earlier age have a higher risk for developing fibroids. Estrogen and progesterone are not produced until a woman starts her periods. So, a woman who started her periods younger is exposed to estrogen for a longer time and has a higher risk.

Pregnancy
Studies have shown that women who have more pregnancies are less likely to have fibroids. This association likely involves a combination of hormonal and non-hormonal factors. When a woman is pregnant, she is protected from exposure to the hormonal fluctuations of her menstrual cycles for 9 months. Women who are older when they have their first baby have an increased risk of fibroids. Delivering a baby causes changes in hormone levels, growth factors, and the way cells respond to hormones. These changes may be protective against fibroids. Pregnancies that do not reach full term do not influence the risk of fibroids.

In women who have had children, breast feeding has a protective effect against fibroids. This finding is likely related to the fact that breast feeding suppresses the ovarian hormones. Interestingly, this protective effect has not been found in black women, possibly because the protective effect is small compared to the other increased risk factors they have.

In some women with fibroids during early pregnancy, an ultrasound after delivery often shows shrinkage or disappearance of the fibroids. At three to six months after delivery, fibroids have disappeared in 36% of women. The cause for this finding may be due to poor blood flow to the fibroids during birth and to normal reshaping of the uterus after delivery.

Age of Menopause

When a woman goes through menopause, her ovaries stop making estrogen and progesterone. So naturally, the later a woman goes through menopause, the longer she is exposed to estrogen and the higher her risk of fibroids is. Usually, fibroids stop growing and shrink after menopause. The average age at menopause is 51.

Hormone Medications

Taking hormone replacement therapy after menopause increases the risk of fibroid growth, whether they are taken as a combination of estrogen and progesterone or just estrogen alone. In these medications, there is a higher ratio of estrogen to progesterone.

Birth control pills have no effect on fibroid risk, regardless of the types of hormones, strength, dose, length of use, or how recently they were used. These medications have a higher proportion of progesterone.

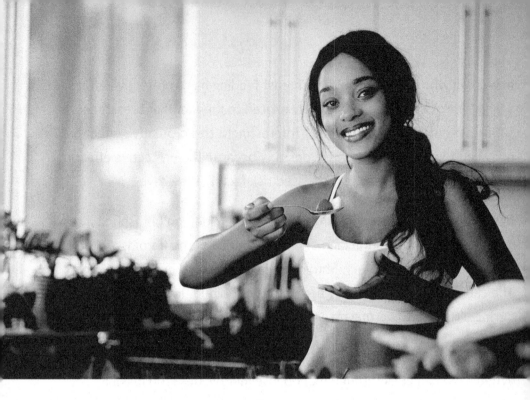

Exercise

Physical exercise decreases fibroid risk. There is some evidence that exercise prevents new fibroids from forming more than it keeps existing fibroids from growing. Women who engage in moderate-intensity physical activity at work have a significantly lower risk of developing fibroids.

Diet

It's very difficult to separate the effects of diet on fibroid risk because racial and cultural difference in diet confuse the data. For example, African American women eat less fruits and vegetables than white women, and they have more fibroids. It's challenging to determine if the difference in fibroid rate is due to the dietary differences or to racial and genetic differences. Accepting this limitation, there is evidence that several dietary risk factors exist.

A diet high in beef, ham, or other red meat increases the risk of fibroids. This has been shown to be true without consideration of the hormones to which the animals have been exposed.

Lower intake of fruits, green vegetables, and fish are associated with higher risk of fibroids. On the other hand, women who eat more fruit and vegetables have a reduced risk of fibroids.

Women who eat a lot of citrus fruits, like oranges and grapefruit, have a much lower risk of fibroids.

There is a lower incidence of fibroids in women who consume a lot of dairy products. This association may be related to levels of Vitamin D.

There is conflicting evidence about the risk associated with soy products. Some studies show them to increase the risk of fibroids, while other studies show them to be protective. A consensus has not yet been determined about the relationship of soy products and fibroids.

Alcohol

Alcohol increases the risk of fibroids. The correlation is stronger for beer than for wine.

Excess Weight

Women who are overweight or obese have an increased risk of fibroids. Because fat cells produce estrogen, it makes sense that women who have an overabundance of fat cells also have an overabundance of estrogen. In overweight women, the risk of fibroids is increased by up to 47%.

Vitamin D

Vitamin D deficiency is a risk factor for fibroids in both black and white women. Women with adequate levels of Vitamin D have a lower risk of fibroids. The higher incidence of Vitamin D deficiency in black women likely contributes to the racial differences in fibroid occurrence.

Vitamin A

There have been studies that show higher levels of Vitamin A are correlated with a higher risk of fibroids. But another study has shown higher levels of Vitamin A are correlated with a lower risk of fibroids as long as the vitamin comes from animal products rather than a vegetarian diet. This suggests a more complex relationship than is currently understood.

Stress

Believe it or not, stress is a risk factor for fibroids because it changes our hormonal balance. Cortisol, a major stress hormone, is regulated by the hypothalamus and pituitary gland, which also regulate estrogen and progesterone. Data on this topic is absent for white women. In studies of black women, those with high-intensity stress levels have a higher risk of fibroids. In particular, fibroids are more common in women who have experienced stress related to racial discrimination. It is possible that the increased risk in this group is related to other factors such as alcohol, diet, and obesity. A correlation between fibroids and stress, depression, or anxiety was not found in Asian women.

Polycystic Ovary Syndrome (PCOS)

Women with PCOS have been shown to have a 65% increased risk of fibroids. Lack of ovulation in women with PCOS leads to continuous high levels of estrogen, promoting fibroid growth. This association may also be due to increased levels of another female hormone, luteinizing hormone (LH) in women with PCOS.

Genetics

Alterations in several genes on the X chromosome have been linked to fibroids. There has been one altered gene (MED12) identified in up to 85% of fibroids, but a direct cause-and-effect link between this gene and the formation of fibroids has not been found. Multiple fibroids from the same woman may have different genetic changes. Several factors related to the DNA, RNA, and receptors on fibroid cells have been identified that seem to play a part in signaling the fibroid cells to keep reproducing or live when they're supposed to die. Genetic alterations have been found in black women, white women, and Asian women. There is not enough information to map out exactly how genetics plays a role in fibroid formation, but clearly the genes are involved.

Environmental Exposures

Several common chemicals have been found to increase the risk of fibroids, presumably because they simulate estrogen-like hormones in the body.

Women whose mothers took diethylstilbestrol (DES) have an increased risk of uterine fibroids. DES is a synthetic estrogen that was given to pregnant women from 1940 to 1971 to reduce the risk of pregnancy complications. Its use was stopped when it was found to cause an unusual vaginal cancer in the daughters of women who took it. Since then, an increased risk of fibroids in the daughters of women who took it, as well as several other risks, have been found.

Animal studies have shown an increased risk of fibroids after *in utero* exposure to bisphenol A (BPA), a chemical in plastic that has been used since the 1960s. Plastic containing BPA is commonly used to make food containers and water bottles. An association between BPA exposure and fibroids has not yet been shown in women.

Women with exposure to phthalates have an increased risk of fibroids. Phthalates are a type of chemicals that have been used in plastics and other materials since the 1930s. They can be found in food packaging, receipt paper, medical devices, medications, toys, and building materials. They're also found in products commonly used by women, including cosmetics and personal care items like lotion, perfume, and nail polish.

Women who have used hair relaxer have a 17% increased risk of fibroids compared with women who never have.

Studies of women who survived the atomic explosion in Japan demonstrate a clear dose-dependent correlation between exposure to radiation and fibroids.

Hair Relaxer

Women who have used hair relaxer have a 17% increased risk of fibroids compared with women who never have. The risk is increased further depending on how many years a woman has used it, how many times per year she uses it, and how many scalp burns she's had. It's interesting to note that hair relaxers contain phthalates, just as many plastics do.

Infections

Pelvic inflammatory disease is associated with an increased risk of fibroids. The higher the number of episodes a woman has had, the greater her fibroid risk. Chagas disease, a tropical disease caused by a parasite, is associated with an increased risk of fibroids. Chlamydia infection may increase the risk as well. There is no correlation between fibroids and genital herpes or human papilloma virus (HPV).

High Blood Pressure

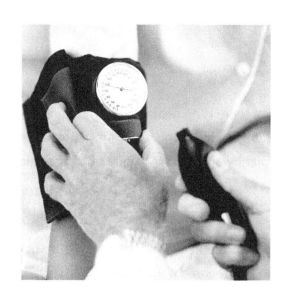

Women with high blood pressure have an increased risk of fibroids. The longer a woman has had hypertension, the greater her risk.

Diabetes

Women who have diabetes have been found to have a lower risk of fibroids. This relationship is not well understood. Since fibroids require a rich blood supply, the overall worsened vascular status in women with diabetes may play a role.

Smoking

Women who smoke have a lower risk of fibroids. As with diabetic women, the impaired vascular status in smokers may play a role.

Factors That Do Not Affect the Risk of Fibroids

At last, some good news! These items have been studied and shown to have no correlation to the likelihood of fibroids.

- Caffeine / Coffee
- Carotenoids
- Fiber
- Folate
- Lycopene
- Vitamin B12
- Vitamin B6
- Vitamin C
- Vitamin E

So, there is no need to skip your morning coffee if you are in a high-risk category for fibroids. Given what else we know about fibroid risk, you might want to have a juicy citrus fruit along with it.

The Three Types of Fibroids

Some complex terms will follow but stick with me. I'm sure you will want to be prepared if your doctor brings up some of this terminology when you seek treatment. Knowledge is power, right? So, here's the scoop.

Fibroids are classified depending on their position in relation to the wall of the uterus. The three types of fibroids are submucosal, intramural, and subserosal.

The inside lining of the uterus is called the endometrium. Just as the inside lining of the mouth is called the mucosa, the endometrium can be thought of as the mucosal layer of the uterus. Submucosal fibroids are positioned so that they touch the endometrium. Whether just a small portion of a fibroid touches a small portion of the endometrium or nearly an entire fibroid pushes into the inside cavity of the uterus, entirely coated with endometrium, this is a submucosal type of fibroid. Uncommonly, an entire fibroid can be on a stalk inside the uterine cavity, like a mushroom cap. These fibroids are called pedunculated submucosal fibroids. They are also sometime called intrauterine or intracavitary fibroids.

The outside lining of the uterus is called the serosa. So, a fibroid that abuts the outside lining is called a subserosal fibroid. It is common for fibroids to distort the contour of the uterus by pushing the serosa outward as it grows. These fibroids can come to look like lumps or knobs on the surface of the uterus. When this happens, they are called exophytic fibroids. Uncommonly, a fibroid can grow on a stalk on the outside surface of the uterus. These fibroids are called pedunculated exophytic fibroids.

Intramural fibroids are positioned within the wall of the uterus. If it is large enough, an intramural fibroid may have portions that are also submucosal and/or subserosal.

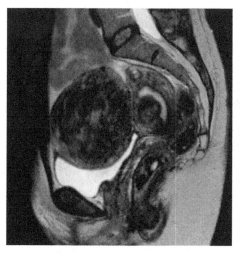 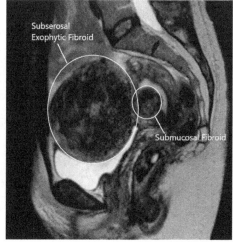

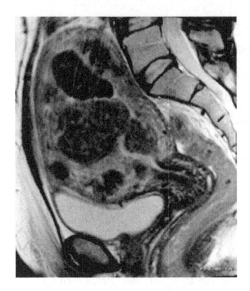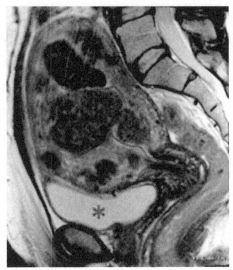

Multiple fibroids pressing against the endometrium, indicated by the curved line running through the uterus. The asterisk marks the bladder.

Symptoms of Fibroids

The majority of women with fibroids actually have no symptoms at all. Many don't even know they have fibroids. However, a wide variety of difficulties can be caused by fibroids. Sometimes a woman may have just one symptom, but often the fibroids manifest as a complex collection of problems.

The symptoms that accompany fibroids are usually related to the location of the fibroids and what they are touching or pushing against.

Heavy Bleeding / Spotting / Clotting

Heavy menstrual bleeding is the most common symptom of fibroids. Submucosal fibroids can irritate the endometrial lining, which is the portion of the uterus that is expelled and bleeds each month. The irritation can lead to heavy, prolonged bleeding. During a period, a woman's body produces an anti-coagulant, a chemical to keep the menstrual blood from clotting. When the bleeding is rapid enough, there's not enough time for the anti-coagulant to work, so a woman may pass clots. Irritation of the endometrium by fibroids may also cause spotting between periods or ongoing

Heavy menstrual bleeding is the most common symptom of fibroids.

continual bleeding. In some women, even if there are not submucosal fibroids, increased menstrual flow has been shown to be associated with intramural or subserosal fibroids.

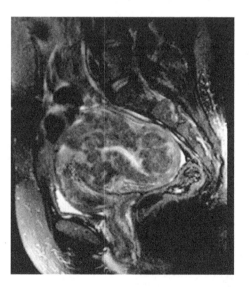 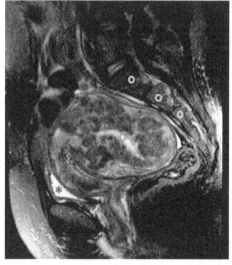

The uterus with multiple intramural fibroids pressing against the spine and sacrum. The uterus is folded back on itself (retroflexed) and is outlined. The bladder is indicated by an asterisk. The diamond marks the endometrium. The circles mark segments of the sacrum at the bottom of the spine.

Pelvic Pain / Cramps / Pressure

Each month, if a woman isn't pregnant, prostaglandins that cause the uterus to contract are produced by the endometrium. These contractions help expel the thickened endometrium, but they also cause cramping. There are other chemicals involved as well that contribute to menstrual cramps, inflammation and the sensation of pressure. Evidence is emerging that the nature of the fibrous connective tissue between the muscle cells is involved in the increased severity of pain in women with fibroids, but the way the process works is unknown. Large fibroids or fibroids that that push adjacent organs out of their normal position can create a sense of pressure in the pelvis.

Urinary Frequency / Urinary Urgency / Urinary Retention

If a fibroid is pressing on the bladder, it can increase the pressure in the bladder, causing urinary frequency and urgency. In some women, the

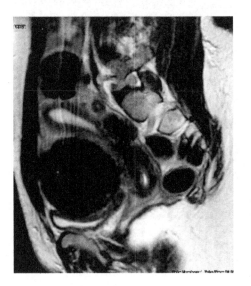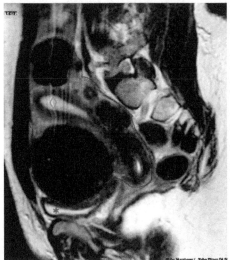

A large fibroid pressing on top of the bladder, which is indicated by the asterisk. The enlarged uterus is outlined, and the diamond indicates the endometrium.

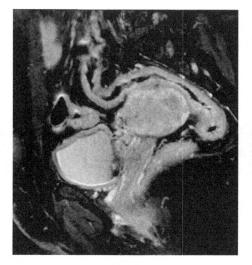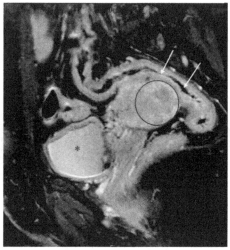

A fibroid, which is circled, pressing against the rectum, indicated by arrows. The bladder is marked with an asterisk.

increased bladder pressure can cause urinary incontinence, especially during sneezing, coughing, laughing, or other activities that increase the abdominal pressure. Sometimes the positioning of one or multiple fibroids within the uterus causes it to shift so that the whole uterus is pressing on the bladder. If a fibroid or the uterus presses against the bladder in just the right way, it can narrow the connection of the bladder to the urethra, making it difficult or impossible for a woman to urinate.

Constipation / Diarrhea / Bloating

If a fibroid is pressing against the lower part of the colon or against the rectum, it can narrow the intestine enough that it is difficult for stool or even gas to pass through. This can cause various bowel symptoms, including constipation, diarrhea, and bloating.

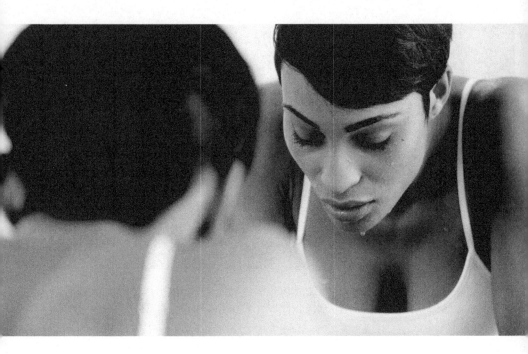

Back Pain / Sciatica

If a fibroid presses against the spine or the nerve plexus in the pelvis, it can cause back pain or pain radiating down the legs.

Pain During Sex

A sense of pain deep in the pelvis during intercourse is more common in women with fibroids. Having multiple or large fibroids doesn't really affect the degree of pain, but fibroids that are located near the top of the uterus tend to be more likely to cause pain than fibroids elsewhere in the uterus.[4]

Infertility / Miscarriage

The vast majority of women with fibroids are able to become pregnant, carry the pregnancy to term, and deliver a normal, healthy baby. The presence of fibroids does not automatically cause an increased risk of miscarriage.[5] Yet, problems with fertility may arise in a several situations.

If the uterus is very enlarged by fibroids, the ovaries may be pushed away from the fallopian tubes, making it less likely for an egg to be able to enter the tube.

If fibroids block the opening of the fallopian tubes, the egg may not be able to reach the uterus. If the fibroids draw enough blood flow away from the endometrium, it may not thicken enough to support a pregnancy, which could result in an early miscarriage. Fibroids that distort the uterine cavity can cause infertility or miscarriage.[6] If there are multiple fibroids or large fibroids, they may impair the ability of the uterus to stretch and enlarge as the fetus grows. These issues could lead to miscarriage later in pregnancy.

The vast majority of women with fibroids are able to become pregnant, carry the pregnancy to term, and deliver a normal, healthy baby.

If you are reading this book, it is likely that you are having some combination of these symptoms. If you are, there is hope! Next, we will delve into what you can do if you are diagnosed with fibroids.

Chapter 3

COMMON NON-SURGICAL TREATMENTS OPTIONS FOR FIBROIDS

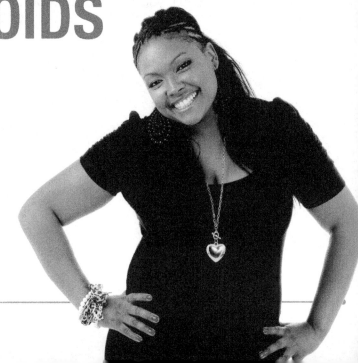

*I*f you are diagnosed with fibroids, you might be wondering what you should do next. The great news is that medical science has truly evolved when it comes to treating the uterus. It's good that you are a modern girl living in a modern world!

If a woman's fibroids don't bother her, for the most part, there's no need to treat them. A basic principle in the practice of medicine is that if a patient is already fine, a medical treatment is not likely to make her better.

An exception to this principle is in the scenario of finding large fibroids in a young woman, particularly in a young African American woman. In this case, treatment may be suggested even if the fibroids are asymptomatic. It's safe to assume the fibroids will continue to grow and will eventually cause problems. By the time they become symptomatic, treatment may require a more complex, challenging, and risky approach.

In describing the various treatment options for fibroids, I'm going to begin with what is least invasive and end with treatments that are most invasive.

Natural Treatments

There are several natural approaches to treating fibroids. They can be divided into the categories of Chinese medicines, homeopathic medicines, and herbal preparations. Most of these preparations are available for sale online, however, you should always consult with an experienced practitioner before using them. Be sure to discuss the risks of becoming pregnant while taking these preparations since they may have adverse effects on pregnancy.

Chinese Medicines

There is very limited information available in the medical literature about traditional Chinese medicines for fibroids. Of all the natural treatments available, however, a few have scientific evidence that supports their efficacy. Compared with a conventional pharmaceutical treatment commonly used in Europe, the herb Tripterygium wilfordii extract, better known as Thunder God Vine, produces a greater reduction in the size of women's fibroids and of the uterus. Combining this same pharmaceutical with Guizhi Fuling formula, also known as Cinnamon Twig and Poria Pill, produces a greater reduction in the size of the fibroids, size of the uterus, and menstrual pain than use of the pharmaceutical alone. No difference was found between the effect of Nona Roguy and one of the most common pharmaceutical fibroid treatments used in the United States. Each of these Chinese medicines is used for an average of three to six months, and none of them produces adverse effects.[7]

Homeopathic Medicines

Practitioners of homeopathic medicine claim success in managing the symptoms of fibroids as well as dissolving them. There is no scientific data to support or refute these claims. For those who are interested in the homeopathic medicines to be used for fibroids, here is a list of several different compounds and the types of symptoms for which they are routinely prescribed.

COMPOUND	SYMPTOM
Ammonium Carbonicum	clotting, profuse bleeding, black blood, thigh pain
Aurum Metalicum Natronatum	fibroids and depression
Belladonna	fibroids and pain with bright red gushing flow
Calcarea Carbonica	overweight, heavy or long periods, cold feet
Calcarea Fluorica	very large, hard fibroids
China Officinalis	heavy bleeding with anemia
Cinchona Officinalis	fibroids with anemia
Erigeron Canadensis	fibroids and urinary frequency
Ferrum Metallicum	heavy bleeding with anemia, pale or watery bleeding
Ferrum Phosphoricum	fibroids with anemia
Fraxinus Americana	foot cramps or feeling of bearing down during cycle
Ipecacuanha	fibroids with heavy bleeding
Kali Carbonicum	prolonged bleeding and back pain
Sabina Officinalis	heavy bright red blood and clots
Sepia Officinalis	dragging pelvic pressure with weariness, painful intercourse
Thlaspi Bursa Pastoris	frequent periods, cramps, back pain, prolonged bleeding
Trillium Pendulum	fibroids and back pain, fainting from heavy periods
Ustilago Maydis	heavy bleeding, clotting, cramps, dark stringy blood

Herbal Preparations

The use of herbal preparations for the treatment of fibroids and their symptoms also is not addressed in the medical literature. For those interested in the commonly prescribed herbs for fibroid symptoms, here is the list.

HERBS TO AID ESTROGEN METABOLISM	
Dandelion	Yellow dock
Milk thistle	

HERBS TO SHRINK UTERINE FIBROIDS	
Chasteberry tincture	Motherwort
Black cohosh	Oleander extract
Dong quai	Red clover
Goldenseal	Red raspberry
Licorice root	Siberian ginseng

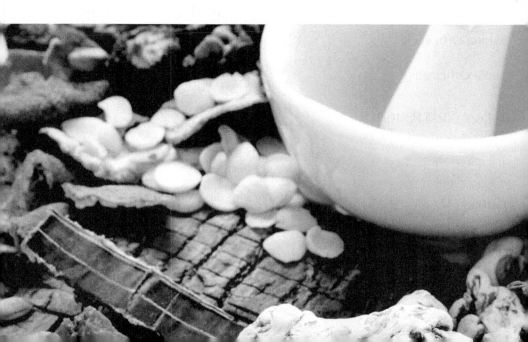

Medical Treatments

Traditional medicine also has remedies to offer, as follows.

Non-Steroidal Anti-Inflammatory Drugs (NSAIDs)

NSAIDs are commonly used to treat the cramping pain associated with menstruation and fibroids. They block the production of prostaglandins, thereby blocking the inflammatory process and uterine contractions responsible for cramps. The most common NSAIDs are aspirin, ibuprofen, and naproxen.

Oral Contraceptives

Oral contraceptives contain either a combination of estrogen and progesterone or progesterone alone. They can be used to regulate the menstrual cycle in an effort to stop spotting between periods or continual bleeding. They can also sometimes reduce the volume of menstrual flow. Oral contraceptives will not shrink the fibroids, however. They also carry several risks, including venous blood clots, stroke, heart attack, liver tumors, gallstones, and mood swings. The risks are much higher in older women and women who smoke.[8]

Leuprolide

Leuprolide is a gonadotropic releasing hormone analogue (GnRH-a). Gonadotropin releasing hormone causes the pituitary gland to release hormones that are involved in the menstrual cycle and pregnancy. When medicine similar to GnRH, called a GnRH analogue, is given long term, it causes the pituitary gland to switch off, so that it no longer produces any menstrual or pregnancy hormones. This mimics menopause and switches off the production of estrogen by the ovaries. The lack of estrogen allows the fibroids to shrink. They can shrink up to 70% after six months of therapy.

A GnRH analogue is often given as a long-acting injection. The most common brand used in the USA is Lupron or Lupron Depot. The downside of using GnRH-a for management of fibroids is that there are unpleasant side effects in up to 95% of women, including hot flashes, decreased libido, vaginal dryness, irritability, and mood swings. Small amounts of other hormones may be given when a woman is taking leuprolide to help manage the symptoms. When the leuprolide is stopped, the fibroids rapidly return to their original size and the fibroid symptoms recur.

Tranexamic Acid

Tranexamic acid is used to stop excessive bleeding. In the presence of bleeding, small clots naturally develop at the point of blood loss to minimize bleeding. Natural systems in the body also break down those blood clots. Tranexamic acid prevents the breakdown of the blood clots formed to stop excess bleeding.

The brand name of tranexamic acid is Lysteda. It is taken as a pill for up to 5 days during the menstrual cycle. It has been shown to decrease menstrual flow by up to 50% and significantly improve women's quality of life.[9] The most common side effects are headache, back pain, and nausea. The medication does not improve menstrual cramping or shrink the fibroids.

Ulipristal

Ulipristal is a selective progesterone receptor modulator (SPRM) that mimics some effects of progesterone on the uterus and blocks others. It results in significant reduction of menstrual flow, decreased cramping, and shrinkage of fibroids. The most common side effects are headache and breast tenderness. The medication does not produce menopausal symptoms, but it stimulates overgrowth of the endometrium. Therefore, it is given for repeated three-month courses, allowing a normal menstrual cycle between each course.[10] Ulipristal is in the process of applying for approval from the Federal Drug Administration in the USA and may soon be used here for fibroids. It is already widely used in other countries.

Medicated Intrauterine Device (IUD)

An IUD is a small device that is inserted into the uterus through the cervix by a gynecologist to prevent pregnancy. Some brands of IUDs contain progestin hormone medication to increase the contraceptive effectiveness. Tiny amounts of the hormone are released every day. In addition to preventing pregnancy, the hormones released from these devices can affect the symptoms from fibroids. They can decrease menstrual flow and cramping. The medicated IUDs can be effective for three to five years depending on the brand. The brands of hormonal IUDs available in the USA are Mirena, Skyla, Liletta, and Kyleena. The Mirena is the most commonly used.

> In addition to preventing pregnancy, the hormones released from these devices can affect the symptoms from fibroids. They can decrease menstrual flow and cramping.

There are a few drawbacks to using a medicated IUD to manage fibroid symptoms. The device may be very difficult to insert in a woman with fibroids, especially if they are submucosal. In women with fibroids, the device is more likely to be expelled from the uterus. The fibroids usually do not shrink when a woman uses an IUD. Also, rarely the hormones can induce similar side effects as oral contraceptives or GnRH analogues. And some women simply do not want a foreign body in their uterus.

Endometrial Ablation

Endometrial ablation is a procedure performed to destroy the endometrial lining inside the uterus. As the endometrium heals, it scars over and leaves less normal endometrial tissue to bleed in the future. Periods usually become very light or completely stop after an ablation. The procedure is moderately painful and is usually performed with sedation or anesthesia.

Endometrial ablation has been available as a treatment for heavy periods for about 20 years and has undergone changes over the years to make it simpler and more effective.

Who Is a Candidate for Endometrial Ablation?

Endometrial ablation is performed for women with heavy menstrual bleeding who have not been helped by treatment with medicines. In certain situations, endometrial ablation should not be performed. Women who want to get pregnant in the future should not have an ablation since pregnancy is likely to be impossible afterwards. A pregnancy that occurs after an ablation has a high risk of complications and miscarriage. A woman who has had an ablation is advised to never get pregnant afterwards.

If endometrial pre-cancer or cancer is suspected, ablation should not be performed. A current pelvic infection or IUD in the uterus are other reasons endometrial ablation should not be performed. Also, if a woman has had a Cesarean section or surgery in the wall of the uterus, like myomectomy, ablation may not be advisable.

It's very common for the uterus to fold on itself towards the front (called anteflexed uterus) or towards the back (retroflexed uterus). Some women are born with the uterus shaped differently than normal. In these situations, it can be very difficult to get some types of ablation devices to pass all the way into the uterus to perform the ablation. The same problem of placing the ablation probe may happen if the inside of the uterus is distorted by fibroids. The size, shape, and position of the uterus are important in making the decision about whether an endometrial ablation should be performed, and if so, which technique should be used.

Technique

An endometrial ablation is performed by placing an instrument into the uterus through the cervix. Local anesthesia is injected into the nerves around the cervix. First the cervix is dilated or stretched open a little bit by passing a thin tube through it, then progressively thicker tubes are inserted. Then the ablation instrument is put in. The instrument is used to destroy the endometrium using one of several different technologies.[11] The procedure may be performed using light sedation, but because the procedure can be painful, many patients choose to have the ablation performed under general anesthesia.

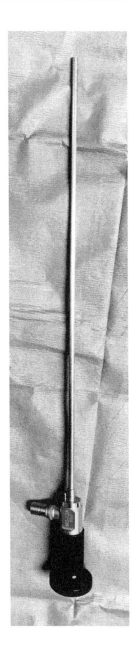

Hysteroscope image courtesy of Kelli R. Beingesser, MD, FACOG.

Hydrothermal Ablation (Genesys HTA)

In hydrothermal ablation, a thin tube with a camera and light on the end of it called a hysteroscope is put into the uterus through the cervix.

Room-temperature saline is instilled into the uterus, and the gynecologist can examine the endometrium through the hysteroscope. The saline is slowly heated up to 90° Celsius (194° Fahrenheit) and allowed to stay inside the uterus for 10 minutes, giving time for the endometrium to burn. The hot fluid is then withdrawn through the hysteroscope to prevent burns to the external structures. The entire procedure usually takes just under a half hour. After ablation using heated fluid, 68% of women return to normal or light bleeding, and 35% stop having periods completely.

Heated Balloon (ThermaChoice)

When using the heated balloon technique, a tube with a soft balloon at the tip is passed through the cervix into the uterus. The balloon is inflated with fluid that is then heated to 87° Celsius. The balloon is left inflated for eight minutes. Since the balloon is soft, as it expands, it takes on the shape of the inside of the uterus, so it's touching all the endometrium. The heated fluid burns the endometrium. The balloon is then deflated and withdrawn. After balloon ablation of the endometrium, 44% of women have light bleeding, and 37% stop having periods.

Laser Ablation

During laser endometrial ablation, a laser fiber is passed through a hysteroscope into the uterus. The laser is turned on and passed across the endometrium until the entire surface is burned. After laser endometrial ablation, 69% of women have light periods, and 39% stop having periods.

Electrosurgery

Electrosurgery is performed through a hysteroscope placed through the cervix into the uterus. There is a wire loop, roller ball, or other configuration on the tip of the electrosurgery device that is heated with electricity to destroy the endometrial lining. The success rates of electrosurgical ablation are similar to the other techniques.

Radiofrequency (NovaSure and Minerva)

During radiofrequency ablation, a thin tube is inserted through the cervix into the uterus. With the NovaSure device, a metallic mesh membrane is collapsed around the end of the tube. The mesh is released and opens like a fan to fill the triangle shape inside of the uterus. A vacuum is turned on to suck the endometrium against the mesh. Then radio waves are run through the metal mesh to heat it up and burn the endometrium.

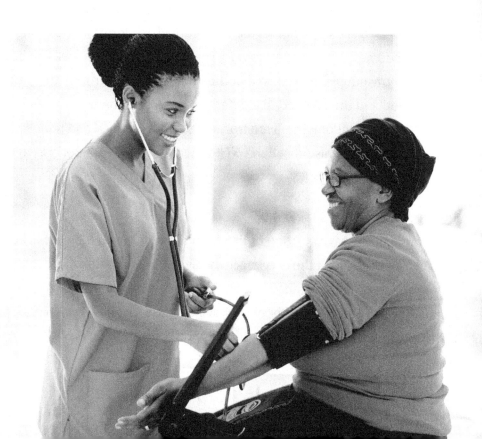

The current is allowed to run for 90 seconds to two minutes. When the ablation is completed, the mesh membrane is re-collapsed around the tube and withdrawn. After this procedure, 78% of women have light or normal menstrual bleeding, and 36% entirely stop having periods.

With the Minerva device, a triangular membrane containing a heating array is opened and fills the inside of the uterus. The membrane is heated until the ablation is completed. The membrane is collapsed, and the tube is removed. The procedure usually takes three minutes to complete. After the Minerva procedure, 93% of women have light or normal menstrual bleeding, and 72% entirely stop having periods.

Freezing Ablation

Ablation of the endometrium by freezing it is performed by placing a thin tube into the uterus through the cervix. Ultrasound imaging is used to guide the placement of the tube. The tip of the tube is cooled to - 60° Celsius (-76° Fahrenheit). As the tip is cooled, ice forms in the tissue of the endometrium and uterine wall. The size of the frozen area can be seen with ultrasound. Once an area of the endometrium is frozen, the probe is warmed and then moved to a different area inside the uterus. When all the areas of the endometrium are frozen, the tip is warmed and removed from the body. After this procedure, 67% of women have light periods, and 22% stop having periods.

Microwave Ablation

During microwave ablation of the endometrium, a thin tube is placed into the uterus through the cervix. Microwave energy is passed through the device to ablate the endometrium. The procedure usually takes 3 to 5 minutes to complete. After microwave ablation, 35% of women have light periods, and 61% stop having periods.

Risks of Endometrial Ablation

As with all procedures, bleeding and infections are possible. Other risks include the small chance of puncturing the uterus and injuring the cervix. If fluid is being instilled into the uterus, it is possible to have it be absorbed by the body and cause fluid overload. There is also a risk of a delayed consequence called "post-ablation syndrome." It can cause pain and ultimately lead to hysterectomy.

What to Expect after Endometrial Ablation

After the procedure, there usually is mild to moderate cramping in the uterus, similar to menstrual cramps. The cramps are usually controlled with NSAIDS like ibuprofen. The cramping may go on for two to three days. Sometimes the doctor will prescribe stronger pain medication for a few days.

There is usually light bleeding or watery discharge that may last from a few days to a few weeks. Just like skin getting burned, the endometrial tissue tends to weep fluid. Women should not use tampons for two to four weeks after an ablation to minimize the risk of infection. Refraining from sexual intercourse for two to four weeks is also recommended.

It is fine to resume exercise the day following the procedure.

While some women are able to return to normal activities and work the day after an ablation procedure, some require two to five days for the cramping to subside.

MRI Guided Focused Ultrasound (MRgFUS)

MRgFUS is a relatively new treatment for uterine fibroids. During this procedure, a woman lies on her stomach in an MRI machine that has high energy ultrasound equipment built in. The MRI imaging can localize the fibroids and other structures in the pelvis. The imaging is used to focus an ultrasound beam on the area of the fibroids while avoiding the structures around the uterus that must not be injured. The focused ultrasound beam heats up small areas at a time of the fibroid tissue until most or all of it has been treated and dies.

The benefits of MRgFUS are that it provides a non-invasive way to treat fibroids, it does not require hospitalization, and women can usually return to normal activities within a few days of the procedure.

There are several downsides to the procedure, however. If there are intestines in the way between the front of the pelvis and the uterus, the procedure cannot be done because of the risk of injuring the intestines. If a woman has large or multiple fibroids, MRgFUS is not a good choice because the volume of tissue that can be eliminated is limited. A fibroid

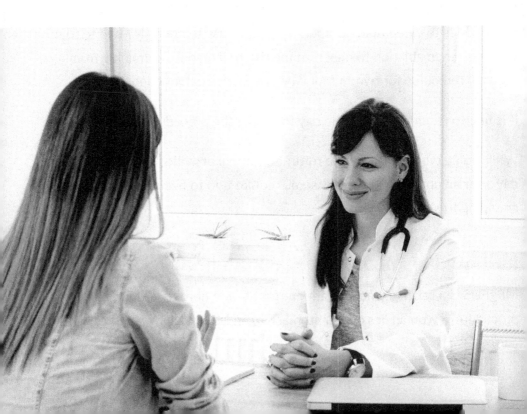

on the surface of the uterus may not be able to be treated because of the risk of heating up structures around the uterus. If a woman has a scar in the uterus from a prior Cesarean section or myomectomy, passing the ultrasound beam through the weakened tissue may damage the uterus. Several women have had babies after MRgFUS, but there is not enough data to determine whether pregnancy is safe after the procedure, so it is usually not performed on women who still want to get pregnant. There are a few other rare risks, including burns on the skin where the ultrasound beam enters the body, damage to structures around the uterus, and temporary back pain.

The benefits of MRgFUS are that it provides a non-invasive way to treat fibroids, it does not require hospitalization, and women can usually return to normal activities within a few days of the procedure.

Because of these concerns, the insurance industry in the United States has decided not to pay for MRgFUS. Because it is an expensive procedure, the lack of insurance coverage practically eliminates it as an option for treatment. There are a few academic institutions with the equipment and the ability to perform the procedure, likely related to research studies. It is also being performed in other countries, including in Asia and South America.

Chapter 4

UFE: A GREAT OPTION FOR MINIMALLY INVASIVE FIBROID TREATMENT

*U*terine fibroid embolization (UFE) has emerged as a highly effective, minimally invasive procedure performed to treat uterine fibroids. It has been a boon to women with significant fibroid symptoms who might otherwise face more serious, fully surgical treatments such as myomectomy or hysterectomy.

Unlike most other fibroid treatments, which are performed by gynecologists, UFE is performed by doctors called interventional radiologists. These doctors perform minimally invasive image-guided surgeries. Just like the procedures performed by cardiologists in the heart, like angioplasty and stent placement, interventional radiologists perform the same techniques in all the other blood vessels outside the heart and use similar catheter-based techniques in all the other organs.

The benefits of UFE for women with fibroids were discovered quite accidentally.

In the early- and mid-1990s, interventional radiologists began collaborating with obstetricians to help minimize life-threatening hemorrhage in pregnant women with abnormalities of the placenta. If the placenta is positioned over the cervix or if it grows into or through the wall of the uterus, there can be massive blood loss during delivery. When imaging technology with ultrasound and MRI advanced to the point that the placenta could be evaluated, obstetricians had advanced warning of these cases. Interventional radiologists could thread a tiny tube or catheter through the blood vessels into the blood supply to the uterus and placenta. A tube would be placed on each side of the uterus, and the blood

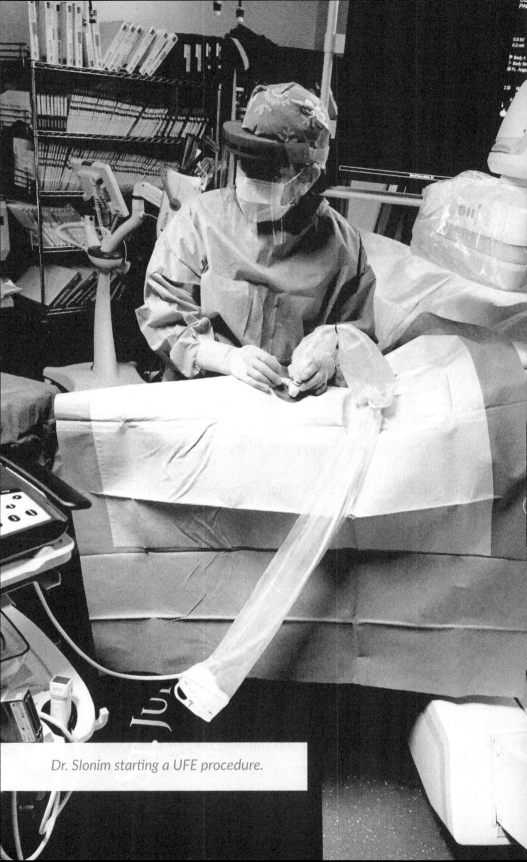

Dr. Slonim starting a UFE procedure.

flow would be plugged to allow safe delivery of the baby and either safe hysterectomy before the woman bled to death or even preservation of the uterus.

As more of these emergency procedures were performed, it was noticed that in women who had fibroids, the fibroids would shrink after the procedure. Eventually, it became clear that blocking the blood flow in the uterine arteries would cut off the blood supply to the fibroids and cause them to die and shrink. Eureka! A new treatment for fibroids was discovered.

The UFE Technique

UFE is usually performed in a hospital. Some outpatient facilities are designed to have all the equipment and safety features necessary for UFE. Many women are excited to be able to go home the same day of treatment. If you have a UFE performed in a hospital, however, they may have you stay overnight.

Since the procedure is performed with sedation or anesthesia, nothing can be eaten or drunk for eight hours beforehand.

When a woman reports for the procedure, she is asked to disrobe and put on a gown. An IV is placed, and blood work is often drawn. Usually there will have been a formal consultation with the doctor before the day of the procedure. During this visit, the doctor will have explained the procedure as well as the risks, benefits, and alternatives to UFE. On the morning of the procedure, the woman will have an opportunity to ask last-minute questions. The nurse will review what will happen during the procedure, fill out necessary paperwork, and have the patient sign a consent form. Often, a urinary catheter will be placed in the bladder to keep it empty and out of the way during the UFE. Sometimes this happens in the pre-procedure holding area and other times it happens in the procedure room after the woman is asleep.

Once everything is ready, the woman will be taken into the procedure room and positioned on the procedure table. There will be a big machine in the room to allow fluoroscopy (moving x-ray) imaging during the procedure. Other people in the procedure room will usually include someone to operate the x-ray equipment, a nurse or anesthesiologist, and a scrub assistant to help the doctor.

When the patient is positioned on the procedure table, the nurse will apply monitors and the x-ray technologist will start sterilizing the area of skin where the doctor will be working. A sterile drape will be positioned to keep everything clean and sterile. Once the monitors are applied the nurse or anesthesiologist will start giving medication through the IV to put the patient to sleep.

After the patient has been put to sleep, the doctor will numb up the area where the tube will be placed, usually with lidocaine. A small puncture into the artery will be made, and a sheath will be placed into the artery. The sheath allows the doctor to thread in the catheter used for the embolization. Watching with the fluoroscopy, the doctor will thread the catheter through the blood vessels right to one of the uterine arteries. Contrast material (dye) will be injected into the blood vessels to localize exactly where the catheter needs to be positioned.

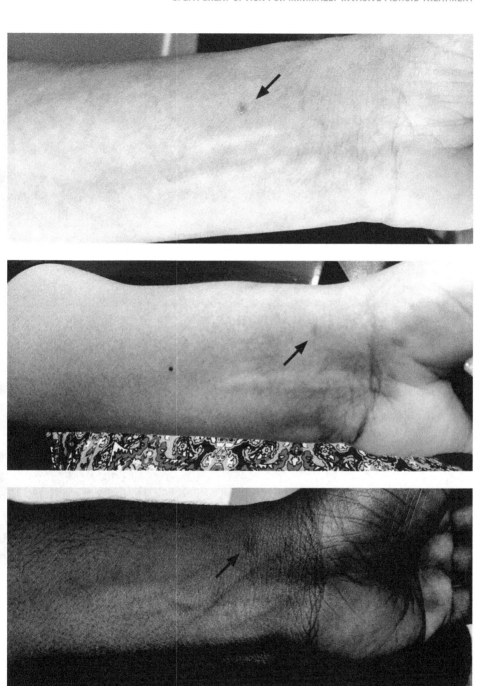

Arrows point to the tiny scar from the uterine fibroid embolization puncture.

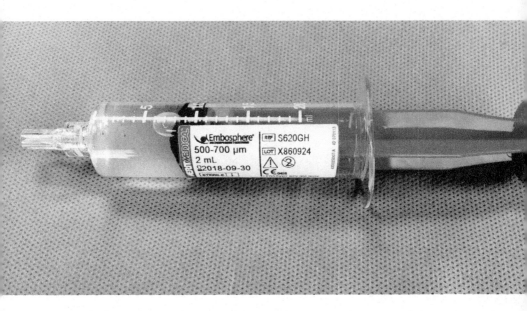

Embosphere particles made by Merit Medical are the most commonly used for UFE in the United States.

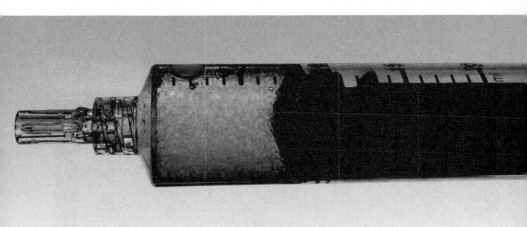

Holding the syringe up to the light makes it easier to see the tiny particles used for UFE.

Once the catheter is positioned in the uterine artery at the appropriate location, tiny particles will be injected into the uterine artery. There are several types of particle commonly used for UFE.

The particles are made of synthetic polymers or gelatin, and doctors can get them in various sizes. The sizes that are commonly used for UFE range from 300 to 1000 microns. To give you an idea of how big this is, a human red blood cell is 7 microns. When the particles are injected into the uterine artery, the blood flow carries them forward into the fibroids. They travel further and further into the smaller and smaller arteries in the fibroids until the blood vessels are too small to let the particles pass. The particles lodge in these tiny fibroid arteries and plug them. Once the artery is plugged, no more blood can get in. When all the tiny arteries in the fibroid are plugged, the blood supply is cut off. With no blood supply, the fibroids will die and shrink.

In very rare cases, there may be additional blood supply to the fibroids from the ovarian arteries or other variant arteries. There are a few other rare variants of the arterial anatomy of the uterus. There may be only one uterine artery supplying the entire uterus. The doctor can usually recognize this situation because injecting the one artery causes the entire uterus to light up. In other cases, the doctor may find only one uterine artery that lights up only half the uterus. In this situation, there will be a search to find another source of blood flow to the uterus, either from the ovarian arteries or from other pelvic arteries. If the variant artery cannot be found, the procedure will not be able to be completed. The patient will usually need another special test, computed tomography angiography (CTA) to localize the variant blood supply to the uterus. Once the vessel is localized, the UFE can be completed in another procedure.

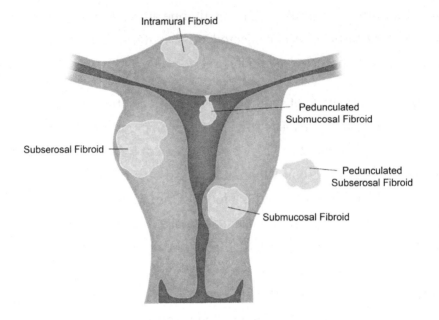

Types of Fibroids

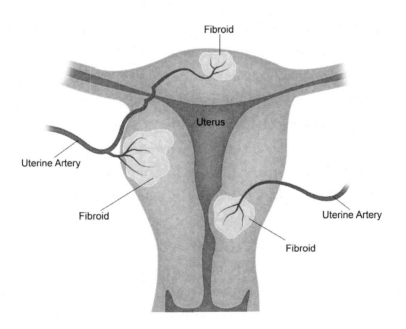

Fibroid Blood Supply

After treating one of the uterine arteries, the doctor will reposition the catheter into the other uterine artery. The injection of particles will be repeated, cutting off the blood supply to the fibroids from both sides of the uterus. In the vast majority of women, the blood supply to every single fibroid comes from one of these two blood vessels. It doesn't matter how many fibroids a woman has. Blocking the flow in these two blood vessels will kill every single fibroid.

When both uterine arteries are blocked, the catheter will be removed. If the puncture was at the left wrist, a band will be placed around the wrist that will hold pressure over the puncture site. The band is usually left in place for up to two hours. With a wrist puncture, the patient can sit up, move around, lie on her side, or curl up to get more comfortable. If the puncture was at the groin, the doctor may use a small plug at the puncture site to seal the hole. If a plug is used, the patient will have to lie flat on her back for two hours without moving the leg. If a plug is not used, the doctor or technologist will hold pressure over the puncture site for about 15 minutes. Then the patient will have to lie flat and still for six hours.

The patient will be taken to the recovery area for observation during at least part of the two- to six-hour waiting period. If the procedure is done in a hospital, she likely will stay overnight. She'll be taken to her hospital room when the recovery nurses feel comfortable that she is stable. If the procedure is done in an outpatient center, she will be able to go home when the waiting period is finished. She will need someone to drive her home.

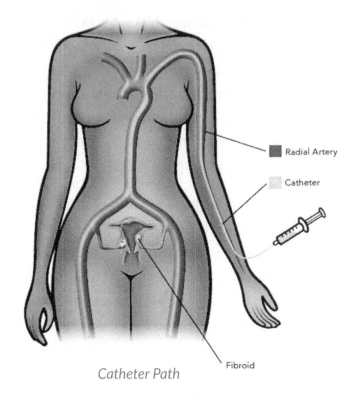

Radial Artery

Catheter

Fibroid

Catheter Path

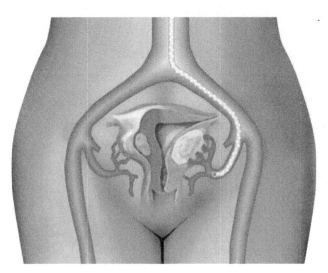

Catheter in Uterine Artery

Are There Risks to Having UFE Treatment?

There are a few risks associated with UFE, all of them quite rare.

There is a small risk of bleeding at the puncture site. At the wrist, this risk is minimal since the blood vessel is just under the skin and very easy to control just by putting a little pressure over the puncture site. The risk of bleeding is higher at the groin, about 5%, because the vessel is deeper. The puncture site can be harder to control there, especially in heavy people. It takes a lot more pressure to stop bleeding at the groin than at the wrist. If a device is used to seal the puncture site, the risk of bleeding is reduced.

Some people can be allergic to the contrast material used during the procedure. The allergic reactions can range from mild to life-threatening. The mild reactions can involve itchy eyes and a runny nose, like seasonal allergies. More severe reactions can cause a skin rash, hives, or swelling in the mouth. The most severe allergic reactions to the dye can cause anaphylaxis. An example of an anaphylaxis-type reaction is when someone who is very allergic to peanuts eats a cookie with a peanut in it: they can die very quickly if they don't get immediate treatment. An anaphylactic allergic reaction can interfere with the heartbeat and blood pressure. It also can cause the airways to narrow, making it very difficult to breath. These severe anaphylactic contrast reactions can occur in 1 in 70,000 cases. It is important to be sure your doctor knows how to manage an allergic reaction if it occurs.

The contrast material is cleared by the kidneys, so it can strain the kidneys or even cause them to fail. If the kidney function is normal to begin with, this risk is negligible. If the patient has any history if kidney problems, the

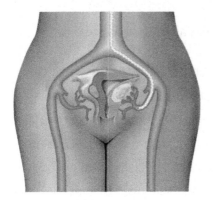 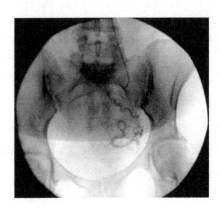

Injection of Dye

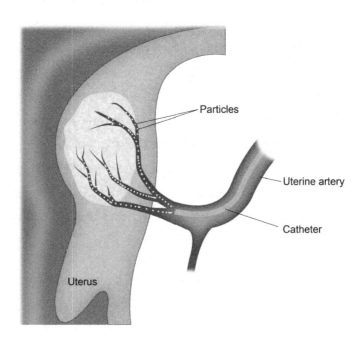

Particles in Uterine Artery

doctor will probably do a blood test to check the kidney function before the procedure to make sure it's safe to give the contrast.

Moving catheters and other instruments around inside the blood vessels could cause damage to blood vessels. Something could get damaged that requires surgery to fix. This risk is extremely rare.

The sedation or anesthesia used to keep the patient comfortable during the procedure can cause problems with the cardiovascular system and breathing. This is true any time a patient is anesthetized for any procedure. To minimize the risks associated with sedation, the heart rate, oxygen levels, and blood pressure are routinely and closely monitored throughout the procedure and recovery period.

When the particles are injected into the uterine arteries, if they flow into unintended blood vessels, they can cause damage to whatever organ's blood flow they block. The areas of greatest concern are the bladder in front of the uterus, the rectum behind the uterus, the vagina, and the gluteal muscles in the butt. In the hands of a skilled interventional radiologist, having particles flow into an unintended blood vessel is extremely rare.

When the blood flow to the fibroids is blocked, it can cause an infection of the uterus. In some cases, the infection could be bad enough that the woman needs a hysterectomy. There have been two cases reported in the medical literature of an infection bad enough that the woman died.[12,13] Neither of those patients were given antibiotics before the UFE procedure. It is currently routine to give antibiotics before UFE, and infections are very rare.

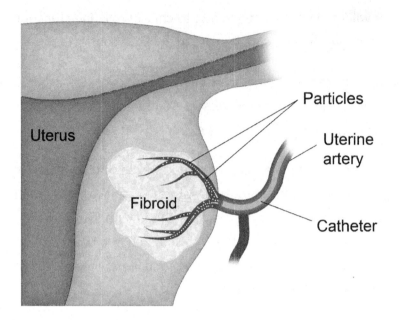

Before UFE

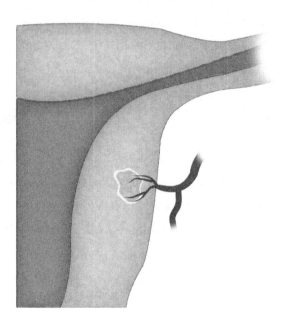

After UFE

Having a UFE may cause an increase in the risk of miscarriage. Several studies have reviewed the pregnancy outcomes after UFE. It is certainly possible for women to conceive, have a normal pregnancy, a normal delivery, and a normal baby after UFE. But there is evidence that the rates of miscarriage and several other problems, including placental abnormalities, pre-term delivery, and post-partum hemorrhage, are higher in women who have had UFE.[14,15] Several studies have compared the pregnancy outcomes after UFE or myomectomy and shown that the miscarriage rate is higher after UFE than after myomectomy.[16,17] For these reasons, myomectomy is considered to be the procedure of choice for women who are considering getting pregnant after fibroid treatment. If you have had children and don't plan to have more, however, UFE is a less-invasive option.

> ... for women who have infertility due to fibroids, having a UFE procedure can increase their likelihood of pregnancy by up to 37%.

On the other hand, for women who have infertility due to fibroids, having a UFE procedure can increase their likelihood of pregnancy by up to 37%.[18] And in some women, there are simply too many fibroids in the uterus to make removal of them safe without risking having to remove the entire uterus. So, for women who are not candidates for surgical myomectomy, for women with multiple fibroids who want to preserve their uterus, or for those who refuse to have surgery, UFE remains a good option. For women who have not practiced birth control for years and have not gotten pregnant because of the fibroids, it is important to be cognizant of the increased likelihood of pregnancy after UFE.

Some women will stop having menstrual cycles after the UFE procedure. This is more common as women get older. Approximately 40% of women

45 years old or older will stop having cycles. Most women welcome the cessation of their cycles, but this could be a big concern if a woman is trying to become pregnant. The lack of cycles usually does not indicate menopause but rather disruption of the normal hormone regulation related to the UFE. Evaluation by a fertility specialist may be necessary to establish where the problem lies. In younger women, the cycles often return spontaneously.

It is possible for a woman to go into early menopause after UFE. Overall, the risk of early menopause is about 2%. It gets higher the closer a woman gets to menopause. Most women go through menopause between the ages of 50 and 55. There have been no studies done to determine the risk of menopause based on the age of the woman having a UFE. I would estimate the risk to be less than 2% for women under age 40, up to 5% for women 40 to 45, up to 15% for women 46 to 50. For women over 50 years old who are still having periods, I usually tell them they have a 50% chance of going into menopause after the UFE procedure.

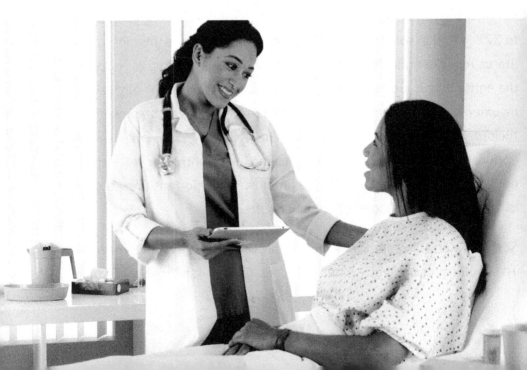

Especially for younger women, it is important to know that it is fairly common for women to have a few hot flashes after the UFE procedure. It does not necessarily mean she is going through menopause. It simply means that the hormone levels have been disrupted by the procedure. The hot flashes usually subside within a week or two.

It is possible to get recurrent fibroids after a uterine fibroid embolization. A woman who makes fibroids will likely continue making fibroids unless there is a significant change in risk factors. There has been no study of the rate of recurrent fibroid symptoms after UFE, but it is likely very similar to the rate after myomectomy. We know that 31% of women between 30 and 40 years old will develop recurrent fibroid symptoms after myomectomy. The recurrence rate rises to 39% for women who had multiple fibroids at the time of myomectomy.[19]

The only difference in the recurrence rate between UFE and myomectomy is that during surgical myomectomy, some of the fibroids may not be able to be removed. Some small, medium, or large fibroids may be left in the uterus if the surgeon cannot reach them or cannot safely remove them without sacrificing the uterus. These remaining live fibroids would continue growing and could cause new symptoms in a relatively short period of time.

After a UFE is performed, every single fibroid will be dead and will shrink. If new fibroids form, they would start the size of one cell and probably would take many years to grow big enough to cause symptoms. For women closer to menopause, it is likely that they would go through menopause before developing new fibroids big enough to cause symptoms.

So, the recurrence rate for fibroid symptoms after UFE is probably a little bit lower than after myomectomy. In my career, I have had two patients return with recurrent fibroid symptoms. In each patient, the symptoms returned about ten years after the UFE. In both patients, we repeated the UFE procedure and the symptoms resolved.

If there is a fibroid mostly within the uterine cavity, especially if it is on a stalk like a mushroom, after the fibroid dies during UFE, it could peel off the wall and get loose in the uterus. Usually in this situation, the fibroid would come out through the cervix, then through the vagina. A woman may find it in her underwear or in the toilet. If this happens, it is not a problem. The problem would be a situation where the fibroid is too big to fit through the cervix. This problem is more likely in women who have never delivered babies, whose cervix has never dilated. If a fibroid is too big to be expelled from the uterus naturally, it can lodge there and cause pain, cramping, and infection. This situation is most likely to occur within a few weeks of the UFE procedure. If a woman develops worsening pain and cramping during this time period, an MRI can be obtained to determine if a fibroid is impacted at the cervix. If so, a gynecologist would need to perform a hysteroscopic myomectomy, which means she would go in through the cervix into the uterus to remove the fibroid. In rare cases where the fibroid is too big to safely remove through the cervix, a hysterectomy may be required.

The MRI exam obtained before the UFE would show if there is a fibroid in a position that may peel off and cause a problem. If a fibroid in this position is small (less than 3 cm or about the size of a walnut), it likely will pass on its own. If it's bigger than that, it would be wise to make sure the patient's gynecologist is willing to remove it if it becomes a problem.

Overall, having a fibroid peel off and pass through the uterus is very rare. In my more than 20 years of practice, I've had only nine patients pass fibroids. They ranged from grape sized to the size of an orange. Most of the women who passed these fibroids either did not feel anything or had a small cramp and some spotting. One of them had very bad cramps, like labor pains. I've had two patients get an impacted fibroid that would not pass, so it is exceptionally rare. In one, her gynecologist removed it through the cervix. In the other, she decided to have a hysterectomy.

Expected Symptoms after UFE

When the blood flow to the uterus is blocked, the body reacts very intensely. The patient develops severe cramping pain, nausea and vomiting, low-grade fever, and malaise. This combination of symptoms is called Post-Embolization Syndrome. Because we know these symptoms are coming, your doctor can take several steps to minimize them. It's unusual to make them go away completely, but an experienced doctor can make them much better than they usually would be.

The pain will be most severe in the first several hours immediately following the procedure. It remains severe the day after the procedure and moderate for up to four days. The pain diminishes with time. Sometimes mild to moderate pain can last up to two weeks in a minority of patients. There are several regimens that may be used for pain control. Usually they include a non-steroidal anti-inflammatory drug (NSAID) and a narcotic medication.

The NSAID will provides pain relief and keep the inflammation caused by the embolization under control. Usually your doctor will want you take it for two weeks to continue treating the inflammation, even if your pain is gone. Various NSAIDs are commonly used, including ketorolac (Toradol), naproxen (Aleve), and ibuprofen (Advil).

Narcotics are very effective for pain relief and are usually used to help treat the pain after UFE. They may be prescribed alone as hydrocodone, hydromorphone (Dilaudid), morphine (MS Contin), or oxycodone (Oxycontin). Other times they are prescribed as combination drugs combined with acetaminophen (Tylenol) or aspirin. These combination drugs include Norco, Lortab, Vicodin, Percocet, Percodan, Roxicet, and Ultracet, among others. As the opioid epidemic spreads, these medications are becoming more restricted but are usually still available to women who have had UFE because of the need to control the severe cramping pain.

Depending on the regimen your doctor puts you on, by two days after the UFE, you may only need take the narcotic medicine for pain that is not controlled by your other medications (breakthrough pain). You will probably only need this medicine for up to five days. Narcotics can cause nausea or an upset stomach, so if you know you have a sensitive stomach, let your doctor know. It helps to take each dose with a little food to protect it from irritation.

If a combination narcotic/acetaminophen drug has not been prescribed, you may be instructed to take Tylenol to help with pain control.

Some doctors will use a time-released pain patch (fentanyl patch) in addition to the other medications. It is placed on your skin the morning of your procedure. It will not become effective for approximately 24 hours, but it will deliver a continuous low dose narcotic pain medication to you for 72 hours.

If a woman is staying in the hospital overnight, she will usually be given a pain pump that lets her give herself a dose of narcotic pain medication at set minimum intervals. For example, she could push the button on the machine to give herself a dose. A beep from the machine will let her know it's been given. She can push the button again immediately, but it won't give her another dose until the interval time has passed, maybe 15 minutes. No matter how many times she pushes the button, she won't get a dose and she won't hear the beep until the time interval has passed. In addition to the pain pump, oral medications are usually given as well in order to get her ready for the time when the pump will be taken away.

A few doctors offer the option of a long-acting pelvic nerve block. If this is used, the pain will be mild rather than severe until the block wears off. This procedure is usually performed while the patient is sedated during the UFE. It involves positioning a tiny needle through the lower abdomen, just below the belly button, into the area where the nerves run that supply the pelvis. An anesthetic is injected that puts all the nerves in the pelvis to sleep. If the block works the way it is supposed to, the woman should have no pain when she wakes up from the procedure. There may be pressure, but no pain. The type of anesthetic chosen for the nerve block will determine how long the block lasts, but it is usually several hours after the procedure. This is truly miraculous because the worst of the pain usually occurs in the first several hours immediately after the procedure.

It is common to experience nausea and possibly vomiting after UFE. During the procedure you will usually be given medication through your IV to block nausea. Most doctors prescribe an anti-nausea medicine like promethazine (Phenergan) or ondansetron (Zofran) for when you go home. Besides the nausea from post-embolization syndrome, the nausea medicine can be helpful if the narcotic pain medicine upsets your stomach.

A common side effect of the narcotic pain medicines is constipation and excess gas. A stool softener like docusate can help prevent the constipation. For women who get constipated, 15 ml of milk of magnesia twice per day can be helpful. If that doesn't work within a day, other options include prune juice, prune juice mixed with milk of magnesia, tea for constipation, laxative pills, laxative suppositories, or Fleet enemas. Many women have their own recipes to treat constipation, and anything that works is usually fine to use.

An over-the-counter gas remedy can help relieve gas pain. Most women do not need it, but for women who are having problems with bloating and gas, it may help. It is important to drink at least eight glasses of water per day.

If a combination narcotic/acetaminophen drug has not been prescribed, you may be instructed to take Tylenol to help with pain control.

Antibiotics are given through the IV just before or during the procedure. They are also sometimes prescribed after the procedure. These medications may be changed depending on the doctor's preference, the patient's preference, her medical situation, or allergies.

The fever that occurs after UFE is a result of the dying fibroids. It is usually low grade, under 101.5 F (38.6 C). It is usually adequately treated with the NSAID medication or Tylenol prescribed after the UFE. It is important not to take Tylenol or any other pain medications if they have not been specifically prescribed by your doctor to avoid dangerous drug combinations or overdose.

Other Things to Expect after UFE

Diet

It is likely you will not be hungry after the procedure. A clear liquid diet the afternoon and evening of the procedure can help prevent nausea and vomiting. If you do not feel hungry, do not eat. The better your pain is controlled, the less likely you are to have nausea. If your stomach has been upset, when it settles down, start with liquids. As you feel better, you may be able to tolerate solids.

Wait until your body is ready to take in food. You may gradually resume your normal diet and routine medications after the procedure.

Activity

The symptoms after UFE usually do not limit routine, simple daily activities. You will be able to move around and walk normally, climb stairs, shower, and feed yourself. Most doctors give instructions to their patients including these that follow: Do not soak in a tub for three days. Do not lift more than five pounds for three days. Cardio exercise is okay as soon as you feel up to it. Do not drive while you are taking the narcotic pain medications or wearing the pain patch. Do not have sexual intercourse for one week. Do not use tampons for two weeks.

Puncture Site

The arterial puncture site at the left wrist or right groin will have a dressing covering it. You may shower the day after the procedure but try to keep the puncture site covered and dry. If the dressing gets wet, replace it with a clean, dry Band-Aid. You may remove the Band-Aid when the puncture site is sealed. Normally, some bruising at the puncture site occurs. The bruise tends to spread out and change colors from red-purple to yellow-blue-green over several days. This process is the normal way that a small amount of blood under the skin is reabsorbed and should not alarm you. There is often a peanut-sized nodule under the skin at the groin puncture site. This is related to the plug used to help seal the puncture. It will slowly resolve over several months. If you notice any rapid swelling or bleeding from the puncture site, you should use direct pressure by placing your fingers and a clean cloth over the site. Immediately call for assistance, report to the nearest emergency room for evaluation, and notify your doctor. Delayed bleeding at the puncture site is very rare, occurring in less than 1 in 500 patients. You should call your doctor if there is any right leg or left arm pain, weakness, or if your foot or hand becomes cold.

Discharge or Spotting

Many women start spotting on the day of the procedure and spot for several weeks. A brown or reddish vaginal discharge is considered normal. It is best to not use tampons for the two weeks after the procedure;

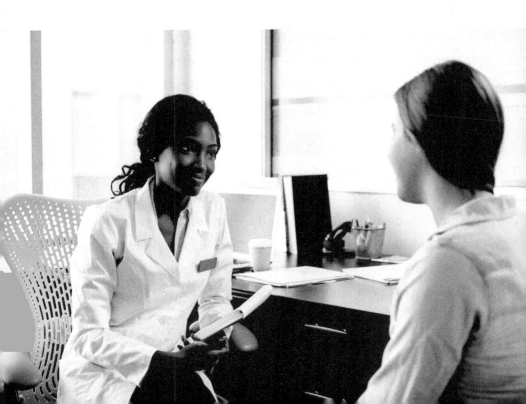

instead use sanitary napkins. Menstrual bleeding may begin just after the procedure and may be irregular. Larger-than-usual blood clots may pass after the procedure, which indicates fibroid degeneration. This is normal and should not be alarming.

Menstrual Periods

Your menstrual periods can be abnormal for three to four months after the procedure. Your first menstrual period may be heavier, lighter, or the same. It may come sooner or later than usual. You may skip a period, or you may have an extra period. If abnormal menstrual bleeding is one of the primary reasons you had the UFE, do not be discouraged. It is quite common that it may take two or three periods before you notice a reduction in the bleeding. The majority of patients will have much lighter periods by the third month after the procedure. Most women, but not all, will have return of periods.

The first and second menstrual periods may be more uncomfortable than typical, although some women notice much less discomfort. Some patients have increased cramps during these periods. These symptoms resolve as the fibroids shrink. As the fibroids shrink and shift, it is common to have intermittent, sharp cramps that come and go quickly for several months after the UFE. They are normal and not a sign of a problem.

The fibroids are going to die in the first two days after the UFE procedure. But it takes three to six months for them to significantly shrink. Therefore, don't expect a rapid relief of pressure, pain, cramping, urinary frequency, and other bulk-related symptoms. But it is very common for patients to report significant improvement as soon as one month after the procedure.

Hormonal Changes

Some patients may experience symptoms because of changes in their hormonal balance after the procedure. Fibroids are driven by estrogen. As the fibroids die, there may be a sudden change in hormones. Some women experience mild depression, which subsides in a few days. Others experience hot flashes and/or night sweats. These symptoms resolve without treatment for most patients.

Return to Work

Most women stay home from work for one week following the procedure. While some women feel ready to resume work as early as three days after UFE, most women do not feel back to normal for up to 10 days. For women whose work requires heavy lifting or prolonged standing, it would be optimal to take an additional week off.

Exercise

You may begin cardio exercise as soon as you feel up to it after the procedure. Any high impact exercise is likely to be quite uncomfortable for one to two weeks. Follow the messages that your body is sending you. If it hurts, don't do it. If you train with weight lifting, do not lift more than 20 pounds for at least two weeks. After two weeks, you may resume your normal routine.

Signs of Potential Problems

Symptoms that might indicate problems include the following:

- Pain that occurs several days or weeks after the initial pain resolved
- A fever several days to weeks after the procedure
- Irregular vaginal discharge, particularly if foul-smelling or profuse
- Vaginal discharge that lasts two months or more

These symptoms may indicate either an infection or partial passage of a fibroid and may require gynecological evaluation. If any of these symptoms occur, contact your doctor so that she can assess the symptoms and make further treatment recommendations.

Gynecologic Care

You should continue your normal gynecologic care. This includes monthly self-breast exams and yearly pelvic exams as suggested by your gynecologist or family practitioner.

Follow-up Care with Your Interventional Radiologist

Your doctor will usually want to see you within a few weeks after the procedure to assess your progress. A repeat MRI may be performed three to six months after the procedure to assure that all the fibroids are dead and to assess their shrinkage.

The Bottom Line

UFE is a great option for women with fibroids who are hoping to avoid invasive surgery. Though there is some recovery time involved, women having UFE usually find that the symptoms are manageable, and the downtime is much less than traditional surgeries.

Chapter 5

SURGICAL OPTIONS FOR FIBROIDS

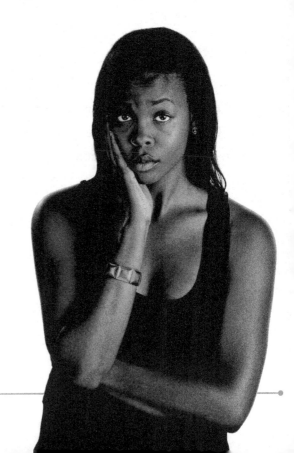

*I*t is my hope that if you are diagnosed with fibroids, you can find a minimally invasive option for treating them. For some women, that doesn't work out. If you do need more extensive surgery, here are some of your options and what you can expect from each of them.

There are two main types of surgeries performed to treat fibroids: myomectomy and hysterectomy. Neither of them is exactly fun but knowing more about them will help you be prepared should you ever need to have them.

Myomectomy

Myomectomy is a surgical procedure in which fibroids are removed from the uterus, but the uterus is left in place. This technique allows a woman to keep her uterus and preserve her ability to become pregnant. It is the procedure of choice for women who need fibroid treatment but still want to have a baby or for women whose fibroids are causing infertility. Myomectomy can be performed many ways, from using minimally invasive techniques to performing surgery that requires a big incision. We are going to discuss all the different types.

Unless it is on a stalk on the outside of the uterus, when a fibroid is cut from the uterus during myomectomy, it usually creates a defect in the muscular wall of the uterus. This defect must be sewn closed and meticulously repaired. With each fibroid removed, there is more damage to the wall of the uterus and more that must be repaired by the gynecologist.

The pre-operative protocol for myomectomy is much the same as for UFE. During an office visit before the day of the procedure, the gynecologist will explain the surgery as well as the risks, benefits, and alternatives to myomectomy. Any necessary blood work is usually performed before the day of the surgery.

Myomectomy is performed in a hospital or surgical center. Because the procedure is performed with anesthesia, nothing can be eaten or drunk for eight hours beforehand.

When a woman reports for the procedure, she is asked to disrobe and put on a gown. An IV is placed. The woman will have an opportunity to ask last-minute questions. The nurse will review what will happen during the surgery, fill out necessary paperwork, and have the patient sign a consent form.

Once everything is ready, the woman will be wheeled into the operating room and positioned on the surgical table. Other people in the procedure room will usually include one or two nurses, the anesthesiologist, and a scrub assistant to help the doctor. The equipment to be used during the procedure will also be in the room.

When the patient is positioned on the surgical table, the anesthesiologist will start giving medication through the IV to put the patient to sleep. After the patient has been put to sleep, a catheter will be placed in the bladder to keep it empty and out of the way during the myomectomy. The steps that happen after this point depend on the specific technique to be performed. There are several different myomectomy techniques that your gynecologist might use.

Hysteroscopic Myomectomy

Fibroids that primarily protrude into the uterine cavity may be able to be removed with hysteroscopic myomectomy. In this procedure, a hysteroscope, a thin tube with a camera on the end, is inserted through the vagina, through the cervix into the uterus. Sterile saline is instilled into the uterus to expand the inside chamber and allow the gynecologist to see the walls better. The fibroid is localized and can then be ground up and removed with an instrument called a hysteroscopic morcellator. Alternatively, pieces of it are shaved off using a wire loop heated with electricity or a laser until it's no longer protruding into the uterus. The pieces that are shaved off flow out of the uterus with the saline. If the fibroid is on a stalk inside the uterus, sometimes just the stalk can be cut, and the fibroid can be pulled out. Hysteroscopic myomectomy may not be possible for very large fibroids.

The recovery time after hysteroscopic myomectomy is usually fast since there is no abdominal incision. Patients are usually able to return to work within two days.

Laparoscopy Assisted Hysteroscopic Myomectomy

Sometimes a thin tube with a light and camera on the end, a laparoscope, is inserted through a small incision in the abdomen to view the uterus from the outside during a hysteroscopic myomectomy. This allows the gynecologist to ensure that the uterus is not perforated or that adjacent organs aren't damaged. This procedure is called laparoscopy assisted hysteroscopic myomectomy. The incision in the abdomen adds a few days of recovery time to the procedure and increases the discomfort and risks.

Laparoscopic Myomectomy

During laparoscopic myomectomy, a laparoscope is placed into the abdomen to guide and perform the surgery. A small incision, about 10 mm, is made in or near the belly button, and the abdomen is inflated with gas. The gas allows instruments to be placed into the abdomen without injuring the internal organs and allows the gynecologist to see. Once the abdomen is inflated, a small plastic tube (port) is positioned through the abdomen to allow the laparoscope to be inserted. The port allows the gynecologist to put instruments in and out without losing access to the inside of abdomen. Two to three additional small incisions (5 to 8 mm) are made, and ports are placed for other surgical instruments to be inserted. Often, the incisions are located low in the pelvis on both sides. The locations of the fibroids determine where the gynecologist decides to place the ports.

Once the laparoscope and instruments are positioned, the gynecologist may take steps to minimize bleeding during the myomectomy procedure. This may be accomplished by injecting medicine around the fibroid that causes the blood vessels to constrict. Putting permanent or temporary clamps on the main arteries supplying blood to the uterus is another technique that can reduce blood loss. Another technique is to wrap a tourniquet around the uterus at the area where the blood vessels enter it. The tourniquet is removed at the end of the surgery.

A newly developing technique involves performing a UFE one to five days before myomectomy to minimize blood loss during the surgery. The gynecologists for whom I've performed pre-myomectomy UFE have been amazed at the small amount of blood loss and therefore the relative ease of surgeries they expected to be very difficult.

At this point, the gynecologist makes an incision in the wall of the uterus and dissects down to the fibroid. The fibroid can then usually be shelled out of the wall of the uterus. The remaining defect in the wall of the uterus must usually be sewn closed.

A small bag is placed through one of the ports into the abdomen, and the fibroid is placed inside the bag. Once inside the bag, the fibroid can be cut into smaller pieces or ground up with an instrument called a morcellator. It can then be removed from the bag through the ports in pieces. Alternatively, a medium sized incision can be made in the lower abdomen to allow removal of the fibroid in one piece. This process is repeated for each fibroid to be removed. If a medium-sized incision is made, it can cause increased pain after the surgery. In rare cases, an incision can be made at the top of the vagina and the fibroid may be removed through the vagina.

The size and number of fibroids that can be removed during laparoscopic myomectomy are determined by the skill and experience of the gynecologic surgeon. A more experienced surgeon will be able to remove more fibroids in a shorter amount of surgical time. In general, the longer the surgery takes, the greater the risk of complications during the procedure there are. And longer surgeries usually involve more blood loss.

Laparoscopic myomectomy requires surgical expertise. Some fibroids may be more difficult to reach or may lie adjacent to internal organs or major blood vessels. For example, fibroids on the back of the uterus may be very difficult or impossible for the laparoscopic surgeon to reach. If she can't get to it, she can't take it out. For this reason, sometimes fibroids are left in the uterus during laparoscopic myomectomy. Alternatively, the surgeon may decide to convert to an open surgery. Up to 28% of laparoscopic myomectomy procedures are converted to an open myomectomy.[20]

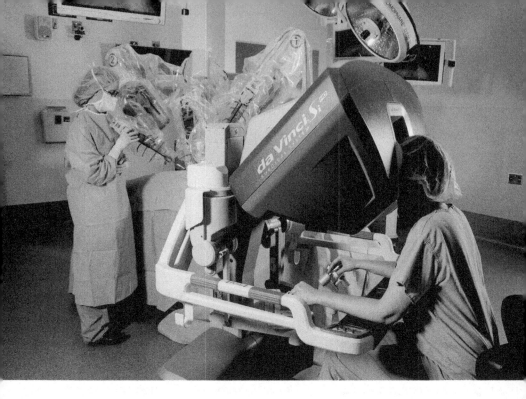

A robotic myomectomy being performed. The surgeon sits at the console while an assistant holds an instrument at the operating table. (©2018 Intuitive Surgical, Inc.)

Laparoscopic myomectomy may take many hours. It is technically more difficult than open myomectomy, but it provides several benefits. These include less pain, less blood loss, a shorter hospital stay, a shorter recovery time, and better cosmetic results. The patient will usually stay in the hospital overnight and be off work for two to four weeks.

Robotic Myomectomy

Robotic surgery is very similar to laparoscopic surgery from the patient's perspective. It involves a few small incisions in the abdomen and pelvis through which ports and instruments are placed. The instruments are attached to a robot, and the surgeon sits at a nearby console to control the robot. It's similar to a console for a video game. The motions of the surgeon at the console are duplicated by the robot.

An important difference between robotic and laparoscopic surgery is that the instruments used by the robot have joints inside the body. They can bend and rotate like a wrist, but the instruments on a laparoscope cannot. This difference makes it easier to suture with the robot than with the laparoscope.

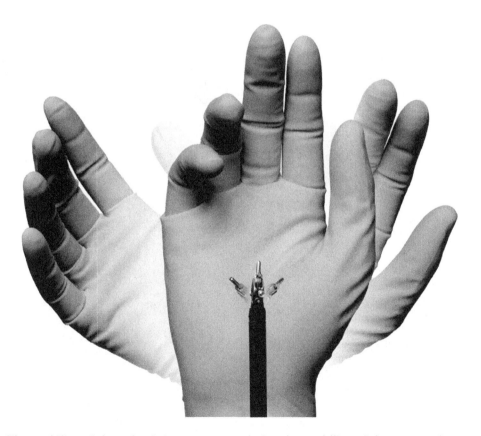

The mobility of the robot's instruments mimics the mobility of the surgeon's hands. ©2018 Intuitive Surgical, Inc.

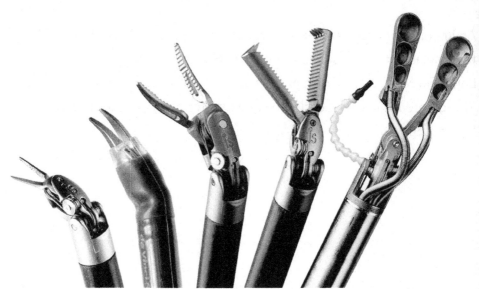

PHOTO CREDIT: INTUITIVE SURGICAL, INC

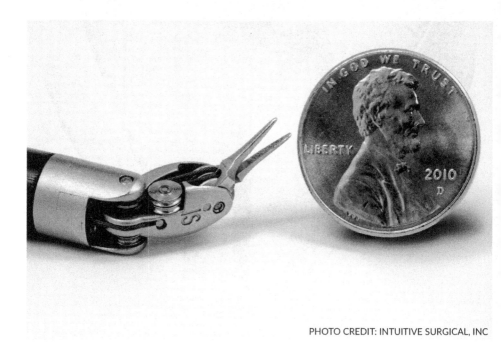

PHOTO CREDIT: INTUITIVE SURGICAL, INC

Surgeons with less experience are able to perform minimally invasive myomectomy with the robot when they may not be able to do so with a laparoscope. Use of the robot decreases blood loss and complication rate, but it significantly increases the time and cost of the procedure. The robot also does not improve the surgeon's access to the back of the uterus. There are similar limitations based on the number and size of the fibroids to be removed. The recovery time after robotic myomectomy is usually the same as after laparoscopic myomectomy, two to four weeks.

Open Myomectomy

In an open myomectomy, an incision is made in the lower abdomen to allow the gynecologist to operate on the uterus directly. There are two different types of incisions that could be made. The preferred approach is to make a horizontal incision very low in the pelvis along the bikini line. Because it follows the natural skin folds, it usually heals better and produces a better cosmetic result. The length of the incision from side to side is determined by how big the fibroids are and how enlarged the uterus is. In some women, the myomectomy can be performed through an incision as short as three to four inches (8 – 10 cm). In women with large fibroids or an enlarged uterus, the incision may need to be longer.

In women with larger fibroids or a uterus that extends above the navel, a vertical incision may be required. This incision is usually made from just below the navel down to just above the pubic bone. It allows the gynecologist to have access to an enlarged uterus in a manner not possible with the bikini line incision. With easier access to the uterus, the surgery can often be performed in a shorter amount of surgical time.

With either type of incision, an open myomectomy often can be performed in a shorter amount of surgical time than during a laparoscopic or robotic procedure. Having open access to the abdomen also allows the gynecologist to get to fibroids along the back of the uterus and areas that may not be accessible with the other techniques.

Comparison of Myomectomy Techniques

There has been a lot of research into whether it is better to perform myomectomy using minimally invasive techniques or open surgery. The data has shown that although the procedure takes longer, a laparoscopic or robotic approach is associated with less blood loss, less post-operative pain, shorter hospital stays, shorter recovery times, and fewer complications.[21,22] A woman with numerous or large fibroids may require an open approach. Otherwise, a minimally invasive myomectomy appears to be a safer technique with an easier and less painful recovery time.

Risks Associated with Myomectomy

The risks of myomectomy depend on the type of surgery performed. In general, the length of surgery correlates with surgical risks. The longer the surgery, the greater the risk of infection, bleeding, anesthesia complications, and other surgical complications.

The risks of hysteroscopic myomectomy include perforation of the uterus, bleeding and infection. The use of antibiotics minimizes the risk of infection. There is a risk of fluid overload due to absorption of the fluid used to expand the uterine cavity during the procedure. Sometimes the surgery must be stopped during the removal of larger fibroids so that fluid overload does not occur. A second procedure is then performed later to remove the remaining portion of the fibroid. There is also a risk that the myomectomy can cause adhesions or scarring in the uterine cavity, making it difficult or impossible to get pregnant in the future.

Laparoscopic and robotic myomectomy require surgical expertise and carry additional risk. Blood loss during surgery is one of the most significant risks. The fibroids have a very rich blood supply and operating to remove them can cause a lot of blood loss. Since women with fibroids lose a lot of blood with their periods and may be anemic to begin with, blood loss during the myomectomy may be more dangerous. Women with a larger uterus tend to have greater blood loss. If a woman is severely anemic before surgery, she may require a blood transfusion prior to surgery. If she loses a lot of blood during the surgery, she may require a transfusion during or after the surgery.

There are several ways to build up a woman's blood count before myomectomy. Taking iron supplements and vitamins can improve iron deficiency anemia caused by menstrual blood loss. Taking hormonal treatment like a gonadotropin releasing hormone analogue (GnRH-a) for several months before surgery can decrease or stop your menstrual blood loss. Although it may cause unpleasant menopause symptoms, it can also shrink your fibroids, making them easier to remove.

During the myomectomy, the several techniques described above may be used by the gynecologist to minimize the bleeding.

Any operation in the abdomen or pelvis can lead to the formation of adhesions. These are bands of scar tissue that form between surfaces inside the abdomen. The adhesions can cause various problems including entangling loops of intestines, blocking fallopian tubes, or causing difficulties during future surgery. The risk of adhesions may be lower with laparoscopic myomectomy than with an open surgery.

If the myomectomy surgery leads to penetration into the cavity of the uterus, scar tissue inside the uterus can form. This can make it difficult or impossible to become pregnant.

A deep incision into the wall of the uterus creates a potential point of weakness. Weakness of the uterine wall could lead to rupture of the uterus during delivery. For this reason, obstetricians recommend delivery by Cesarean section after certain types of myomectomy. For example, Cesarean section may be recommended if the myomectomy involved the full thickness of the uterus into the cavity, if the fibroid was on the top of the uterus (fundal), or if multiple large fibroids were removed. It is also recommended to deliver by Cesarean section if the time between myomectomy and delivery is less than a year. The obstetrician may want to review the surgical records to help determine if a vaginal delivery is safe after the myomectomy.

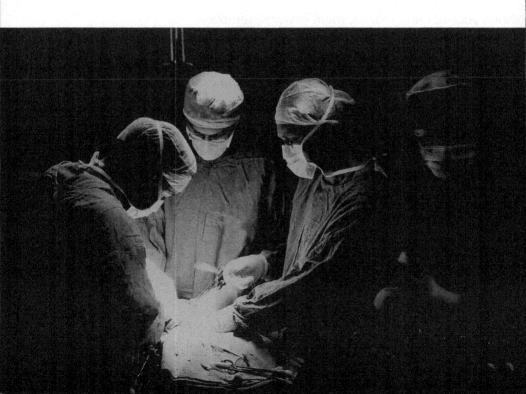

If something unexpected is found, like a cancer, the uterus or ovaries may need to be removed to remove the cancer. If a gynecologist encounters uncontrollable bleeding during a myomectomy, she may have to remove the uterus to save the woman's life.

In extremely rare cases, a gynecologist can operate to remove what she thinks is a fibroid, but it turns out to be a cancer. In this case, if she cuts up the tumor inside the body without containing it, the cancer can spread throughout the abdomen and pelvis. For this reason, the Food and Drug Administration (FDA) has issued a warning about the use of laparoscopic power morcellators without the use of a containment system.[23]

There are other risks of myomectomy that are the same as for any big operation. The surgical anesthesia can cause problems with the cardiovascular system and breathing. The heart rate, oxygen levels, and blood pressure are usually closely monitored throughout the surgery and recovery period. Other forms of monitoring may be used as well to help decrease the anesthesia risks.

Blood clots can form in the legs or pelvis during or after the surgery, causing pain and swelling. If they travel through the veins to the lungs, they are called pulmonary emboli and are fatal 20% of the time. Getting a woman out of bed and walking soon after surgery can help prevent blood clots. Automatic pumping pads that wrap around the legs to squeeze them and compression stockings are also used to prevent blood clots.

Open myomectomy carries the additional risk of wound separation and wound infection, especially in obese patients, smokers, or people with diabetes.

Especially in women with multiple fibroids, there is a risk that all the fibroids may not be amenable to removal. Regardless of the type of myomectomy, there is also the risk of fibroid recurrence. New fibroid symptoms will be seen in 21% of myomectomy patients. In younger women and those with multiple fibroids, the recurrence rate is up to 39%.[24]

What to Expect After Myomectomy

Each gynecologist will have her own set of post procedure instructions. These are some general guidelines to give you an idea of what to expect.

Diet

You will be allowed to eat as soon as your appetite returns after surgery. Nausea and slow bowel recovery are risks after all abdominal surgery. It is a good idea to eat only light meals until you have passed gas.

Activity

You will be required to get out of bed and walk around within a few hours after surgery. This is to minimize the risk of blood clots forming in the veins in your legs or pelvis. It also decreases the risk of pneumonia, constipation, and improves your overall recovery process. Several short walks per day are recommended.

You will be able to shower the day after surgery but taking a bath will not be permitted, usually for a few weeks. Do not lift anything that will make you strain during the four- to six-week recovery period. Vigorous exercise should not be performed until after the recovery period. Do not drive while you are taking the narcotic pain medications.

Do not put anything in your vagina until your doctor says it's okay. This means do not have sexual intercourse, use tampons, or douche. This restriction is usually for two weeks.

Incision Sites

Usually the incision site or sites will be covered with a thin film of sealant glue. Some gynecologists will leave this sealant open to the air while others will cover it with gauze and an adhesive bandage. The small incisions of laparoscopic surgery will be mildly sore. The larger incision of an open surgery will have more pain, including the pain from any tissues that were cut or stretched at the opening. The pain medications will help you manage the discomfort and the pain should get better every day. If you had a transvaginal myomectomy, it usually will be less painful than an abdominal incision. You should call your doctor if your skin develops redness or warmth that expands around the incision, if you develop a high fever, or if cloudy or malodorous drainage from the incision develops.

Discharge or Spotting

Vaginal spotting is common after a myomectomy as you heal. A yellow, brown, pink or red vaginal discharge is considered normal. Call your doctor if you have profuse bleeding or if your discharge is malodorous or looks like pus.

Menstrual Periods

Your menstrual periods can be abnormal for several months after the procedure. Initially, they may be heavier, lighter, or the same. You may skip a period, or you may have an extra period. Most women, but not all, will have return of periods.

The first and second menstrual periods may be more uncomfortable than typical, although some women have much less discomfort with periods after the procedure. Some patients have increased cramps during these periods. These symptoms resolve as the uterus heals.

Relief of pressure, pain, cramping, urinary frequency and other bulk-related symptoms will be noticed as the pain from the surgery subsides.

Pregnancy should be avoided until your doctor advises you it's okay. This can be as early as two months after a myomectomy but may be as long as six months.

Hormonal Changes

Some patients may experience symptoms as a result of changes in their hormonal balance after the surgery. There may be a sudden change in hormone levels. Some women experience mild depression, which subsides in a few days. Others experience hot flashes and/or night sweats. These symptoms resolve without treatment for most patients.

Return to Work

Most women stay home from work for six weeks following open surgery. After robotic or laparoscopic surgery, most women can return to work in up to four weeks. Some women may be able to return to work in as soon as two weeks if their fibroids and incisions were small.

Hysterectomy

Hysterectomy is the most invasive treatment option and since other treatments are available for fibroids, you may never need one. If you do need one, however, you will want to be informed about what to expect. Any surgery that removes an organ is a big deal. Just like myomectomy, a hysterectomy can be performed lots of different ways. We're going to go through them all.

A hysterectomy is a surgery to remove the uterus completely. Over 400,000 hysterectomies are performed each year in the United States alone, mostly for non-cancerous diseases. If a woman is under the age of 40 and a hysterectomy is performed, the ovaries are often left behind if they appear healthy.

> **Hysterectomy is the most invasive treatment option and since other treatments are available for fibroids, you may never need one.**

At this point, I want to clarify a common misunderstanding. Many women believe that if the ovaries are left in the body, it is a "partial" hysterectomy. That is not the case. If the uterus and ovaries are removed, it is called a hysterectomy with an oophorectomy (that's the medical term for removing the ovaries). If the uterus is removed and the ovaries are left in the body, it's called a hysterectomy or total hysterectomy. If the uterus is removed but the cervix is left in place, it's called a partial hysterectomy.

During an office visit before the day of the procedure, the gynecologist will explain the surgery as well as the risks, benefits, and alternatives to hysterectomy. Any necessary blood work is usually performed before the day of the surgery.

A hysterectomy is performed in a hospital or surgical center. Because the procedure is performed with anesthesia, nothing can be eaten or drunk for eight hours beforehand.

When a woman reports for the procedure, she is asked to disrobe and put on a gown. An IV is placed. The woman will have an opportunity to ask last-minute questions. The nurse will review what will happen during the surgery, fill out necessary paperwork, and have the patient sign a consent form.

Once everything is ready, the woman will be wheeled into the operating room and positioned on the surgical table. Other people in the procedure room will usually include one or two nurses, the anesthesiologist, and a scrub assistant to help the doctor. The equipment to be used during the procedure will also be in the room.

When the patient is positioned on the surgical table, the anesthesiologist will start giving medication through the IV to put the patient to sleep. After the patient has been put to sleep, the gynecologist will perform a pelvic exam. When a woman is asleep, all her muscles will relax. She will also not feel pressure or pain. These factors allow the gynecologist to assess the

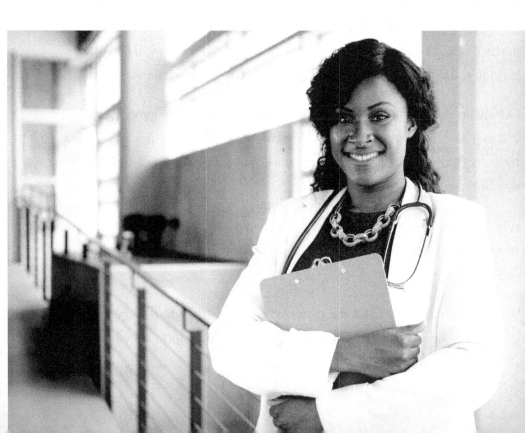

woman's anatomy more thoroughly before making an incision. A urinary catheter will be placed in the bladder to keep it empty and out of the way during the hysterectomy.

During a hysterectomy the lining over the uterus, the connections to other organs, and the ligaments that hold the uterus in place in the pelvis are cut. The blood vessels along both sides of the uterus are cut and closed. Separating the uterus from the other organs and from the pelvis must be performed without damaging the organs and structures next to it. The steps taken to achieve that depend on the specific technique to be performed. The following are the types of hysterectomy that your doctor may advise for you.

Total Abdominal Hysterectomy (TAH)

Total abdominal hysterectomy involves removal of the uterus and cervix through an abdominal incision. Usually, the uterus can be removed through a horizontal incision just above the pubic bone at the bikini line. A vertical incision from the navel to the pubic bone may be performed if the uterus is massively enlarged with fibroids. In extreme cases, an incision is extended above the navel for situations when better visualization may be required. Once the uterus is freed from the adjacent structures, an incision is made from inside the pelvis at the top of the vagina, so the cervix can be removed. The uterus and cervix are removed in one piece. The top of the vagina is usually sewn shut, and the abdomen is then closed. The recovery time after a TAH or "open" hysterectomy is usually six weeks.

Vaginal Hysterectomy (VH)

Vaginal hysterectomy is the removal of the uterus and the cervix through the vagina. A cut is made at the top of the vagina all the way around the cervix to access the inside of the abdominal cavity. Then the uterus is separated from the adjacent structures and blood vessels much like during an open hysterectomy. Once it is freed from the surrounding structures, the uterus and cervix are removed through the vagina. The top of the vagina is then sewn closed. For some women with a uterus enlarged from fibroids or other problems, the uterus may be too large to remove through the vagina. This is particularly true for women who have never had the vagina stretched by delivering a baby. The recovery time after a vaginal hysterectomy is usually two weeks.

Laparoscopy-Assisted Vaginal Hysterectomy (LAVH)

During laparoscopy-assisted vaginal hysterectomy, a laparoscope is placed inside the abdomen while a vaginal hysterectomy is performed. Just like during laparoscopic myomectomy, a small incision is made near the belly button, and the abdomen is inflated with gas. A small plastic tube (port) is positioned through the abdomen to allow the laparoscope to be inserted. The port allows the gynecologist to put instruments in and out without losing access to the inside of the abdomen. Additional small incisions may be made for other surgical instruments to be inserted. Having the scope in the abdomen helps visualization and can aid in the surgery if necessary. Laparoscopic assistance is especially useful in cases where there is scarring, endometriosis, or a mass in the pelvis. The recovery time after LAVH is usually two to four weeks.

Total Laparoscopic Hysterectomy (TLH)

Total laparoscopic hysterectomy is performed almost entirely using a laparoscope. The ports, instruments and laparoscope are inserted into the abdomen with a TLH procedure.

Once the laparoscope and instruments are positioned, the gynecologist performs the same steps as for an open hysterectomy. The uterus is separated from the surrounding structures. A cut in the vagina at the edge of the cervix is made from the inside, and the uterus may be removed through the vagina. The vaginal edges are closed using the laparoscopic instruments. Rather than removing the uterus through the vagina, some gynecologists extend one of the laparoscopic openings to make it just large enough for the uterus to fit through. Unless it is enlarged, the uterus can usually be removed through an incision about four inches long. If one of the port incisions is extended, it can cause increased pain after the surgery.

If the uterus is too large to remove through the vagina, it can be pulled partially into the vagina and cut into smaller pieces or ground up with a morcellator. It can then be removed from the vagina in pieces.

Laparoscopic hysterectomy is technically more difficult than open hysterectomy, but it provides several benefits.[25] These include less pain, less blood loss, a shorter hospital stay, a shorter recovery time, and better cosmetic results. The recovery time after laparoscopic hysterectomy is usually two to four weeks.

Robotic Hysterectomy

During robotic hysterectomy, the uterus and cervix are removed much like during laparoscopic hysterectomy. But as with a robotic myomectomy, the instruments are attached to a robot, and the surgeon sits at a nearby console to control the robot. The combination of high-definition 3D magnification and small instruments that can bend and twist like human hands make the surgery easier. The surgeon can control the robot's movements precisely and can do the surgery in tiny spaces with better visualization than with conventional laparoscopic surgery.

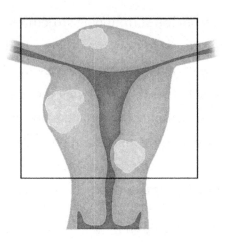

The square roughly indicates the portion of the uterus that would be removed during a supracervical hysterectomy.

Use of the robot decreases blood loss, complication rates, and length of stay in the hospital.[26] The recovery time after robotic hysterectomy is usually the same as after a laparoscopic hysterectomy: two to four weeks.

Supracervical or Subtotal Hysterectomy

Supracervical or subtotal hysterectomy is the removal of the uterus through an abdominal incision, laparoscopically or robotically, leaving the cervix behind. Because the cervix is left in the body, this procedure is also called a partial hysterectomy. During this type of surgery, the uterus is cut just above the cervix and removed. The top of the cervix is sewn closed. The ligaments that attach to the back of the cervix carry nerves that supply the vagina and can affect sexual activities if removed or disturbed.

The advantages of the supracervical hysterectomy may include better sexual function following surgery and better pelvic support. Some believe sexual function is maintained better with this surgery than with traditional TAH because the mucous secreting glands in the cervix continue to produce mucus that reduces vaginal dryness, especially if the ovaries are removed. But many gynecologists disagree with this notion, pointing out that the glands in the lower vagina help more with moisture than those from the cervix. A supracervical laparoscopic hysterectomy takes less time to perform than a total abdominal hysterectomy, which speeds up recovery. There is less post-operative pain, less risk of infection, less risk of bladder or ureter damage, and less risk of bleeding. The rectangular line in the image below encloses the portion that is removed in a supracervical hysterectomy.

There are a few disadvantages of supracervical hysterectomy. The first is that because some of the inside lining of the uterus is usually preserved with the cervix, a woman may continue having a small amount of spotting or light menstrual cycles until she goes through menopause. Leaving the cervix may lead to fibroid recurrence in the cervix. The last disadvantage is much more significant. Leaving the cervix, and possibly a small part of the uterus and endometrium, in place leaves the risk of cervical, uterine, or endometrial cancer. These risks are eliminated during a total hysterectomy. For this reason, most gynecologists will no longer perform a supracervical hysterectomy.

Salpingo-oophorectomy

Salpingo-oophorectomy is the removal of the ovary and the fallopian tube only. Bilateral salpingo-oophorectomy or BSO means that both ovaries and tubes are removed. It can be performed with a hysterectomy and is known as a TAH BSO in the case of an abdominal incision. It is called a TVH BSO if done vaginally. If a woman is pre-menopausal, the ovaries and tubes are usually not removed as long as they look normal to the surgeon. Removal of the ovaries will immediately induce menopause and remove the benefit of the ovarian hormones. There is a 17% increased risk of coronary heart disease after hysterectomy with removal of the ovaries compared with hysterectomy leaving the ovaries in place.[27]

For women who are very close to menopause or in menopause, most gynecologists will recommend removal of the ovaries at the time of hysterectomy. The ovaries will stop producing their hormones once menopause starts. If they are removed, the risk of future ovarian cancer is removed as well.

Risks of Hysterectomy

There are several risks associated with hysterectomy. Just as in any surgery, there is a risk of excessive bleeding that may require transfusion due to anemia or low blood pressure related to excess blood loss. Infections of the abdominal incision, the vaginal cuff, or in the pelvis are the most significant risks. Antibiotics are used before surgery to prevent this but are not always successful. Wound separation can occur with infections and is more common in obese patients, smokers, or people with diabetes. If a wound separates, a delayed closure can be attempted if the incision remains uninfected.

The risks of anesthesia include pneumonia and cardiac problems. In fact, women with underlying serious medical

... women who underwent a hysterectomy at or under the age 35 years had a 4.6-fold increased risk of congestive heart failure and a 2.5-fold increased risk of coronary artery disease...

problems such as heart disease are at risk of a heart attack due to the effects of anesthesia drugs. Other risks of hysterectomy are blood clots that travel to the lung, known as pulmonary emboli, and are fatal 20% of the time. Early walking after surgery and compression stockings are used to prevent blood clots. Blood thinners may be used in high risk individuals such as obese women or those with a history of blood clots.

According to one study, women who underwent a hysterectomy at or under the age 35 years had a 4.6-fold increased risk of congestive heart failure and a 2.5-fold increased risk of coronary artery disease even if the ovaries are left in place.[27]

Bladder, ureter, and bowel complications can occur because they are near the uterus and cervix. A catheter is placed in the bladder before the procedure and removed soon after surgery, but not without discomfort and risk of urinary tract infections. Rarely, women may have the inability to empty the bladder after surgery related to spasm of the urethra. Replacement of the catheter for several days may be required until the spasm resolves.

Recovery after a Hysterectomy

Most women who have a hysterectomy are in the hospital between one and five days. After a vaginal, laparoscopic, or robotic surgery, women usually go home after one to two days. For open surgery, release from the hospital may be delayed by a slow return of normal bowel function. A woman must be able to keep food down before she can be sent home.

Walking soon after surgery is necessary to reduce the risk of blood clots in the legs and encourage prompt bowel function.

There can be significant pain after hysterectomy, more so after an open procedure than after the less invasive surgeries. Narcotics may be required for pain relief and can cause side effects such as nausea, itching, and constipation.

Even if the ovaries are not removed, their blood supply may become reduced because part of their blood supply comes from the uterus and fallopian tubes. The reduced blood supply can result in an earlier than expected menopause. If both ovaries are removed, the woman will go into menopause immediately.

Hormone supplementation may be needed depending on the woman's symptoms.

Sexual changes can occur as a result of low hormones or due to that fact that the nerves to the upper vagina and cervix are removed. Vaginal dryness may also contribute to sexual changes.

It takes a full six to eight weeks after a TAH to be able to return to normal activities such as exercise, lifting, and sexual intercourse.

It takes a full six to eight weeks after a TAH to be able to return to normal activities such as exercise, lifting, and sexual intercourse. LAVH and

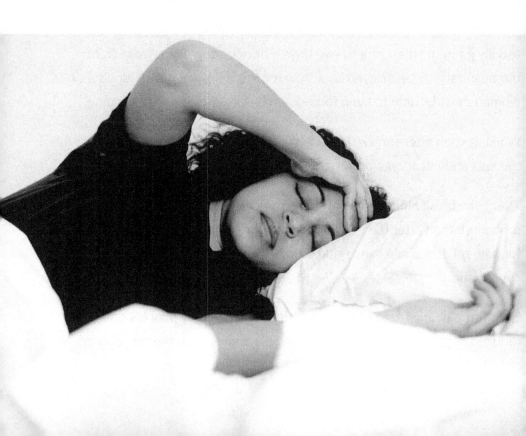

robotic-assisted surgeries only require two weeks of recovery time before resuming normal activities, but sexual intercourse has to wait for six weeks.

Spotting and vaginal discharge can occur after any type of hysterectomy while you recover and in the case of supracervical hysterectomies, spotting can be permanent until menopause.

Chapter 6

NOT FIBROIDS? OTHER POSSIBLE CAUSES OF MISERABLE PERIODS

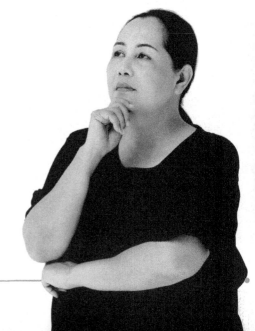

lthough fibroids are common, there are other diagnoses that could be causing your menstrual woes. In this chapter, I will delve into other possible causes for your abnormal bleeding and pain.

Uterine Polyps

Uterine polyps are growths from the inside lining of the uterus known as the endometrium. The endometrium is composed of glands and other tissue. This lining grows each month under the influence of estrogen and progesterone, which are produced by the ovary. During each month's menstrual cycle, the lining is shed if an egg does not become fertilized and is implanted in the endometrium.

A uterine polyp, also known as an endometrial polyp, is made of many endometrial cells that have overgrown in one place. This overgrowth of cells is usually attached to the lining by a stalk like the stalk of a mushroom. Because it's on a stalk, a polyp can move around inside the uterus. Less commonly, they can attach to the lining on a broad base. The polyp has a spongy consistency and has blood vessels in it which makes it subject to bleeding.

Polyps do not grow in the muscular wall of the uterus or hang on the outside of the uterus. Several organs in the body can grow polyps, such as the nasal cavity and the colon. Uterine polyps are the most common reason that women report abnormal uterine bleeding. Polyps can be tiny, smaller than an apple seed, or they can grow quite large, to the size of a lime. If an endometrial polyp has a long enough stalk, it can pass through the cervix into the vagina, though this is rare.

Incidence

Endometrial polyps occur in approximately 8% of women and increase with age. Polyps are rare in women under 30 years old. Over 80% of women with polyps have no symptoms.[28]

In women who have an endometrial polyp, the polyp is found to have cancer or pre-cancer up to 3.4% of the time. A polyp is more likely to be cancerous if there is abnormal bleeding. In women who are in menopause, who are over 60 years old, who have diabetes or high blood pressure, or who are obese, the risk of cancer in the polyp is increased. Of women with polyps, cancerous or precancerous polyps are almost four times more likely in postmenopausal women compared with premenopausal women. Women who take tamoxifen, a medication that affects estrogen and is used to treat breast cancer, have a higher risk of cancer in a polyp, but having breast cancer does not increase the risk. The risk of cancer in a polyp is not affected by the number of pregnancies a woman has had or the size of the polyp. Large polyps are not more likely to have cancer than smaller ones.[29]

If there is bleeding from a polyp, it is more likely to be cancerous, especially in postmenopausal women. In postmenopausal women with a bleeding polyp, the risk that it is cancerous is three times higher than if the polyp is not bleeding.[30]

Causes and Symptoms

The exact cause of uterine polyps is unknown, but hormonal factors play a role in their development. Much like fibroids, polyps respond to estrogen by growing. Any condition that increases estrogen levels or drugs that act like estrogen, such as tamoxifen, can cause endometrial cells to grow and reproduce themselves.

The symptoms of uterine polyps can vary but almost all include bleeding. A polyp can affect menstrual periods, causing them to become heavier. They can last longer or occur more frequently. Sometimes there is spotting between periods, with red or brownish discharge. Some women have spotting after sex. Some women develop bleeding after menopause. Pain has not been reported as a symptom. Polyps can interfere with fertility. Sometimes, polyps go away on their own, and occasionally they fall off their stalk and get flushed with the period or at other times that may go unnoticed, such as during bowel movements.

Diagnosis

Several tests can be performed to diagnose an endometrial polyp. Occasionally, polyps can be seen protruding through the cervical opening at the time of a pap smear.

One imaging test that is often performed when a woman has abnormal uterine bleeding is an ultrasound. When an ultrasound is performed by passing the probe over your lower abdomen, it rarely detects a polyp. More often, the ultrasound shows an area of thickening of the endometrium. If the endometrium looks abnormally thick, usually another test will need to be performed. A better way to evaluate the endometrium is with a transvaginal ultrasound (TVUS). In this examination, an ultrasound probe shaped like a smooth, narrow vibrator will be placed in the vagina. The scanning part is at the tip. With the probe against the cervix, a very good view of the uterus and endometrium can be achieved. Even still, it is rare to be able to see a polyp with ultrasound unless it is very large.

A very effective test to diagnose a uterine polyp is a sonohysterogram, also called a hysterosonogram. In this exam, a speculum is placed in the vagina. A doctor will pass a narrow catheter through the cervix into the uterus. The speculum is removed, and the ultrasound probe is placed in the vagina. While scanning with the probe, saline is injected through the tube into the uterus to expand the cavity. A polyp is then easy to identify as it floats around in the saline.

Another imaging test that can be used to diagnose a polyp is a hysterosalpingogram (HSG). This exam is usually performed if a woman has a history of miscarriages or infertility. With the woman lying on an x-ray table, a speculum is placed in the vagina. The doctor will pass a narrow tube through the cervix into the uterus. While watching with the x-ray, contrast is injected through the tube into the uterus. The doctor will be watching to see if the contrast is able to pass through the fallopian

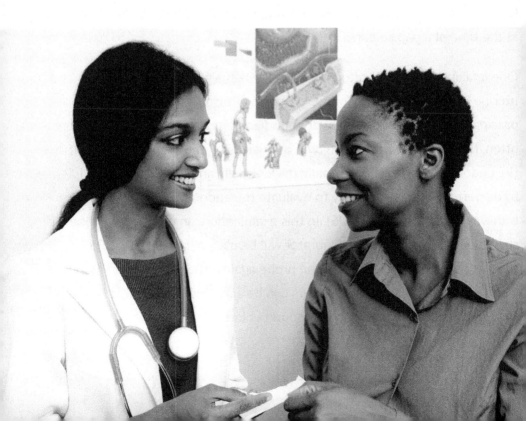

tubes into the pelvis. But if there is a polyp in the uterus, it will look like a smooth structure outlined by the contrast. Often, it can be seen moving around inside the uterine cavity.

The definitive diagnosis of a polyp is made during a hysteroscopy, which is often performed to evaluate abnormal bleeding that has no known cause. Hysteroscopy is an outpatient procedure that can be performed in the office or the hospital. A narrow scope is introduced into the vagina and passed through the cervix into the uterus after the cervix has been dilated. The uterine cavity is filled with saline fluid to allow the gynecologist to see the surfaces. A polyp or other abnormalities can be found this way. Usually, the polyp is removed during the same hysteroscopy procedure during which it is discovered.

Risk Factors

There are several risk factors for the development of uterine polyps. These include increasing age, obesity, high blood pressure, and taking tamoxifen.

Treatment Options

If a woman has no symptoms from a polyp, observation and follow-up is adequate unless she has risk factors for cancer. For polyps that cause symptoms, medications can sometimes be effective. Gonadotrophin-releasing hormone analogue (GnRH-a) or progestins may decrease the symptoms, but they usually resume when the medication is stopped. Polyps that cause symptoms are usually removed through the cervix during hysteroscopy at the time of diagnosis.

Technique for Hysteroscopic Polypectomy

Polypectomy is performed by placing a hysteroscope into the uterus through the cervix. The patient is often instructed to take an NSAID before the procedure. She is usually given light sedation or anesthesia and an injection of local anesthesia into the nerves around the cervix. First the cervix is dilated or stretched open a little bit by passing a thin tube through it, then progressively thicker tubes. Then the hysteroscope is put in and the uterus is inflated with saline for better visualization. The polyp is then removed either with special scissors, a blade, a hysteroscopic morcellator, an electric current, or a laser device. Then the hysteroscope is removed. Polypectomy is generally a very safe procedure, but there are small risks of bleeding, infection, and puncturing the uterus.

What to Expect after Hysteroscopic Polypectomy

After the procedure, there usually is mild to moderate cramping in the uterus, similar to menstrual cramps. These are usually controlled with

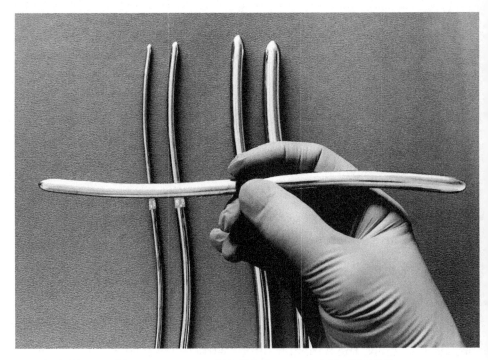

Cervical dilators. Photo courtesy of Kelli Beingesser, MD, FACOG

NSAIDS like ibuprofen. The cramping may go on for two to three days. Sometimes the doctor will prescribe stronger pain medication for a few days.

There is usually light bleeding or spotting that may last for a few days. Women should not use tampons for two to four weeks after a polypectomy to minimize the risk of infection. Refraining from sexual intercourse for two to four weeks is also recommended.

It is fine to resume exercise the day following the procedure, but heavy lifting should be avoided for two weeks.

While some women are able to return to normal activities and work the day after a polypectomy procedure, some require two to five days for the cramping to subside.

Endometriosis

Endometriosis is a disease that results in endometrial (uterine lining) tissue growing in places outside of the uterus such as on the fallopian tubes, ovaries, bladder, bowel, or even distant places like the lung. The cause is unknown, but hereditary factors and the immune system may contribute. The mechanism of this abnormal growth known as endometrial implants is thought to be the result of the backward flow of blood during menstruation. However, 90% of women have this occur each month, so other factors must contribute. Once the lining implants on another surface, it undergoes thickening each month as a result of hormones from the ovaries.

The hormones cause microscopic internal bleeding that causes an inflammatory response, makes tiny blood vessels grow, and causes scar formation that is responsible for the clinical consequences of this disease.[31] While the lining of the uterus can shed each month during menstruation, the endometrial implants have nowhere to go.

Endometriosis is one of the most common and worst diseases seen by gynecologists. Aside from the fact that endometriosis is not cancer and has a low risk of turning into cancer, there is nothing good about this debilitating disease that affects women in the prime of their lives, causing misery and emotional suffering.

When endometriosis is on the ovary, it can cause cysts to form that fill with blood, known as endometriomas or chocolate cysts due to their liquid contents turning brown over time.

The primary symptoms of endometriosis are abdominal or pelvic pain, excruciating periods, and pain during intercourse. The pain is described as

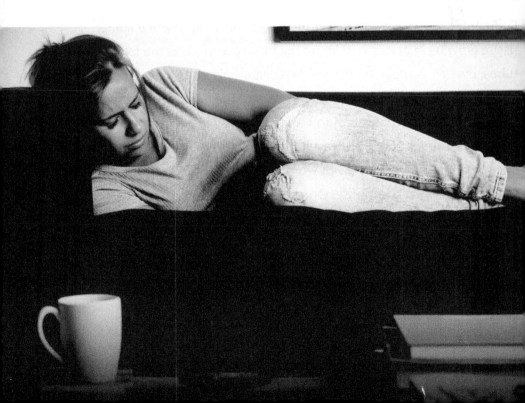

cramping, but can be sharp, cause nausea and vomiting, or cause painful bowel movements. Some women have no symptoms at all. The condition is considered chronic and incurable, but both surgery and medications are helpful in relieving some of the symptoms. Depending on the location, endometriosis can cause infertility, and affected women have a higher risk of premature birth, miscarriage, placental abnormalities, small infants, and Cesarean section.[32]

When seen through a laparoscope, typical implants are blackish-blue, red, white, clear, or yellow.

Incidence or Prevalence

Between 2–50% of women are believed to have "silent" endometriosis while approximately 40-60% who have painful periods beyond the norm have endometriosis. Infertility affects 20-30% of women with endometriosis. Endometriosis is found in 7-10% of US women in the general population, and approximately 4 per 1000 women are hospitalized due to pain from this condition each year.[33] Because laparoscopy diagnoses it, the actual prevalence is unknown. It has been known to regress in 30% of cases but tends to be a progressive disease for most.

Risk Factors

There are multiple risk factors for endometriosis. They include family history of endometriosis, early onset of menstrual periods, short menstrual cycles (less than 27 days between periods), long duration of menstrual flow (more than seven days), heavy bleeding during periods, and delayed childbearing. Conversely, women who have given birth have a reduced risk of endometriosis. Oxygen deficiency and iron deficiency may contribute to the early onset of endometriosis.

Signs and Symptoms

About one third of women with endometriosis have no symptoms. When they do have symptoms, it usually depends on the area involved. The most common symptoms include painful periods, heavy or irregular bleeding, pelvic pain, lower abdominal or back pain, and painful sex. Other common symptoms include pain with bowel movements, often with cycles of diarrhea and constipation, bloating, nausea and vomiting, groin pain, pain with urination and/or urinary frequency, and pain during exercise.[34]

When women have a laparoscopy, the most common sites where endometriosis is found are on the ovaries, behind the uterus next to the rectum, on the broad ligaments (that connect the sides of the uterus to the sides of the pelvis), the ligament behind the cervix that connects it to the sacrum, the rectum and last part of the colon, the bladder, and the ureters that run from the kidneys to the bladder.

Treatment Options for Endometriosis

Medications that disrupt the monthly production of hormones are currently recommended to treat endometriosis. These include gonadotropin-releasing hormone analogues (GnRH-a), progestins, oral contraceptive pills, and androgens. The use of aromatase inhibitors, medicines that block the production of estrogen, is usually for refractory or recurrent endometriosis. Chinese herbal medicine given either by mouth or as an enema has been found to be as useful if not more effective for some endometriosis symptoms compared to some conventional Western medicines. Rectal or lower back pain did not respond better with the Chinese herbs, but they caused fewer side effects.[35]

Birth control pills that stop the periods can be an effective treatment of endometriosis.

The injection of a GnRH-a medication like Lupron works well to reduce endometriosis pain. The pain relief can be long-term (6-12 months) after stopping the injections. Lupron is an expensive drug that induces medical menopause which is reversible. Because of bone loss, hot flashes, and vaginal dryness, only six months of injections are usually recommended. If small amounts of other hormones are given to minimize the side effects when a woman is taking Lupron, it can be used for 12 months.

Birth control pills that stop the periods can be an effective treatment of endometriosis.

Synthetic progestins, including Medroxyprogesterone acetate (Provera) and Megestrol acetate, can be effective for endometriosis pain suppression whether given orally or as an injection.[36,37] There is a longer delay in the return of ovulation with the injectable progestins. Side effects include weight gain, fluid retention, depression, and spotting. A progesterone-containing intrauterine device (IUD) can also be used to suppress menstruation and reduce endometriosis pain.

Danazol is a synthetic steroid that acts to reduce luteinizing hormone (LH) and follicle-stimulating hormone (FSH) production from the pituitary in the brain. It also has a weak androgenic (masculinizing) action. Danazol works well for endometriosis, but due its side effects such as acne and hair growth, other less expensive and equally effective medications are preferred. Danazol takes three to six months to show a positive effect.

Letrozole (Femara) is an aromatase inhibitor that works by blocking the formation of estrogen. It also results in suppression of endometriosis.

Surgery is the only guaranteed way to diagnose endometriosis and can be helpful if removal of the implants is performed at the same time. However, total eradication of all the sites of endometriosis is impossible in most cases. Hysterectomy can offer the best chance for cure and improvement as long as the woman has completed childbearing. Removal of the ovaries at the same time as hysterectomy is recommended due to the recurrence rate of endometriosis if they are left behind, but only if the woman is close to menopause.

Ovarian endometriomas can be drained, or the entire cyst can be removed. Cyst removal by laparoscopy results in better pain relief and pregnancy rates than drainage.

In the case of infertility, removal of implants and scar tissue coupled with medical management offer the most hope for conception. However, the rate of recurrent pain is 44% with surgical management and 53% with medical management.[38,39]

Outlook

Endometriosis cannot be predicted or prevented but it can be managed with variable outcomes. A high index of suspicion is needed, especially if a young woman has trouble with her periods and misses school or other activities as a result of pain and bleeding. The diagnosis can only be made by laparoscopy but using oral contraceptives during this time period might be the best chance to prevent progression and preserve fertility. The long-term safety of oral contraceptives has been established for those without any history of blood clots or other conditions that might predispose to blood clots.

Adenomyosis

Adenomyosis is a common condition that is similar to endometriosis in that portions of the uterine lining are found in places they should not be. In the case of endometriosis, the implants are outside of the uterus. In adenomyosis, the uterine lining forms little pockets inside the muscular wall of the uterus. An inflammatory response occurs, and during the menstrual cycle when estrogen levels surge, these pockets expand and cause a variety of symptoms. Common symptoms include abnormal bleeding, chronic pain throughout the month that acutely worsens during menstruation, and heavy, irregular bleeding. The condition is often underdiagnosed but thought to be present in 20–30% of women.

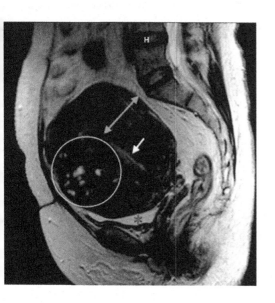

Diffuse thickening of the wall of the uterus by adenomyosis. The single-headed arrow points to the endometrium. The double-headed arrow shows the abnormal thickness of the uterine wall. The asterisk marks the severely compressed bladder. Cysts within the glandular tissue form the bright spots in the uterine wall, which are enclosed by the circle.

The cause of adenomyosis is unknown, but it is thought to be a result of the abnormal infiltration by the endometrium into the muscle portion of the uterus. This infiltration is thought to be due to disruption of the barrier layer between the endometrium and the muscle, called the junctional zone. Other factors are thought to be involved, including high levels of estrogen, an imbalance between estrogen and progesterone, and impaired immunity.[40]

Invasion of the endometrial tissue into the myometrium has been divided into three categories. In the mildest form, the junctional zone is thickened up to 12 mm, either in one area or all throughout the junctional zone. This is termed junctional zone hyperplasia and is considered normal in women of childbearing age. When the junctional zone is thickened more than 12 mm, either in one area or all around the inside of the uterus, it is termed adenomyosis. When there is a mass of the abnormal glandular tissue in the muscle, it is termed an adenomyoma. A uterus with adenomyosis can also have one or several adenomyomas. Adenomyomas can sometimes project off the surface of the uterus or into the uterine cavity.

Risk Factors

There are multiple possible risk factors for adenomyosis, although there is conflicting data about most of them. The risk factors with the most convincing data include multiple pregnancies and births, prior dilatation and curettage (D&C), prior uterine surgery like myomectomy or Cesarean section, and use of medications that influence the menstrual hormones, like tamoxifen and antidepressants.[41] Most women are diagnosed in their 40s or 50s, although MRI has allowed the diagnosis of adenomyosis at younger ages.

Symptoms of Adenomyosis

The common symptom of adenomyosis are very similar to the symptoms of fibroids. They include pelvic pain, severe cramps, a feeling of heaviness in the pelvic region, irregular bleeding, heavy bleeding, painful sex, and chronic pelvic pain. Because of the similarities between these symptoms and the symptoms of fibroids, adenomyosis is often misdiagnosed as fibroids. Even the large adenomyomas can be invisible with ultrasound, so if there are no fibroids present on which to blame the symptoms, some women remain undiagnosed. Eventually, a woman with chronic pelvic pain, heavy bleeding, and no obvious cause undergoes a hysterectomy. When the uterus is studied under the microscope, it is discovered that the woman had adenomyosis.

Diagnosis of Adenomyosis

It can be very difficult to diagnose adenomyosis. It is often confused for fibroids because of the similarities of the symptoms with fibroids. Adenomyosis is usually invisible on ultrasound, even transvaginal ultrasound. Because it is a process that happens in the wall of the uterus, it is not discovered during an endometrial biopsy either. The only imaging study that will discover adenomyosis is a pelvic MRI. MRI is not a common screening test because it is so expensive. So, most women with adenomyosis do not learn the source of their problems until they have a hysterectomy.

Treatment Options for Adenomyosis

Natural Treatments

The natural remedies that are used for adenomyosis are directed at controlling the symptoms of heavy bleeding and cramping rather than directly treating the disease. The treatments include traditional Chinese remedies, herbs, vitamins, massage, yoga, and diet. Staying at your optimum weight is also important because excess estrogen is created in fat cells.[42]

Medications

Conventional medical treatments are often prescribed for adenomyosis and consist of hormones and pain relievers. Progestins are the first-line agents, while oral contraceptives may also be effective. It is best to treat continuously to totally stop monthly menstruation. When the periods stop, the symptoms of adenomyosis stop as well. Non-steroidal anti-inflammatory drugs can help with the pain, but they do not improve the heavy bleeding or feeling of heaviness in the pelvis.

GnRH analogues lead the ovaries to stop making estrogen, which can be a useful strategy. Combination with aromatase inhibitors, medicines that stop the creation of estrogen, helps in reducing the uterine size and symptoms.

Medication-containing intrauterine devices are usually effective in reducing blood loss, uterine size, and painful cramps.

Uterine Artery Embolization

Uterine artery embolization (UAE) is the same technique that is used to block the blood flow to fibroids. When it is performed for adenomyosis, smaller particles are used to target the abnormal glandular tissue. UAE is effective about 75% of the time in relieving the adenomyosis symptoms.[43]

Surgery

Adenomyomectomy is a surgical procedure to remove the adenomyomas while leaving the uterus in place. It is similar to myomectomy for fibroid removal, but it can be more challenging. Adenomyomas are less well defined compared to fibroids, making localization and complete removal difficult or impossible. Pre-operative imaging may improve localization and allow for more complete removal of the abnormal tissue. Sometimes the adenomyomas can be removed using laparoscopic surgery and sometimes open surgery is required. If there is diffuse adenomyosis rather than focal collections of the glandular tissue, removing the abnormal tissue may be impossible without removing the entire uterus.

Hysterectomy is the definitive cure for adenomyosis. If the uterus is not too enlarged, this can be accomplished robotically, laparoscopically or through the vagina. Otherwise, either a horizontal or vertical incision is made in the lower abdomen.

Pelvic Congestion Syndrome

Pelvic congestion syndrome occurs when there are varicose veins in the pelvis around the ovaries and uterus. It can cause chronic dull or aching pelvic pain. Many doctors are unfamiliar with the condition, so it can go undiagnosed for years.

The primary symptom of pelvic congestion syndrome is chronic pelvic pain. The pain is usually worse after standing or sitting for long periods of time, late in the day, during or after sexual intercourse, and just before your periods. It usually feels better when you lie down. Sometimes there is pain on only one side of the pelvis, usually the left side. Other symptoms can include pain during periods, abnormal menstrual bleeding, tenderness over the ovaries, backache, gastrointestinal symptoms, and urinary frequency. Women with pelvic congestion syndrome may also have visible varicose veins on their vulva, buttocks, or legs.

Just like varicose veins in the legs, the pelvic varicose veins are caused by abnormal valves in the veins. The valves are supposed to keep the blood returning to the heart from flowing backwards. When they stop working (called becoming incompetent or insufficient), the blood pools at the lowest point. This causes the veins to swell and expand. It is unknown why the swollen veins cause pelvic pain, and some women with enlarged pelvic veins have no pain or other symptoms.

Risk Factors

There are a few known risk factors for pelvic congestion syndrome. The most common cause is thought to be pregnancy. Women who have had multiple pregnancies are especially prone to it. During pregnancy, the veins dilate to accommodate the increased blood flow to the uterus. Weight gain and shifts in the pelvic organs can sometimes cause the veins to be intermittently obstructed. These changes can lead to long-term valve malfunction.

Hormonal factors are also involved. Conditions that elevate estrogen levels increase the risk because estrogen dilates the veins. After menopause, when the estrogen levels have dropped, the syndrome is very uncommon. Heredity may play a role too. If your mother or sister has pelvic congestion syndrome, you are more likely to have it. Finally, any anatomic condition that causes obstruction of the outflow from the ovarian or other pelvic veins can lead them to dilate and develop valve malfunction.

Diagnosis of Pelvic Congestion Syndrome

It can be very difficult to diagnose pelvic congestion syndrome. The dilated veins cannot be felt during a pelvic exam. On an ultrasound, they may be visible, but lots of women have prominent pelvic vessels without having any symptoms, so they are often ignored. If a CT scan or MRI shows one

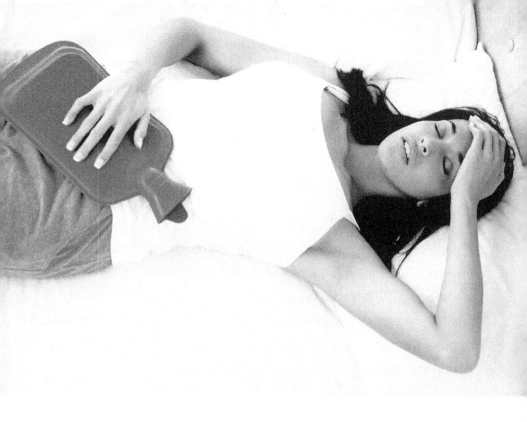

of the ovarian veins to have a diameter of 1 cm, that is certainly abnormal. When a woman is lying down flat, the veins may be decompressed. For this reason, they may also be invisible on CT scan, MRI, or even during laparoscopy. The definitive way to diagnose pelvic congestion syndrome is by injecting x-ray dye into the ovarian veins (performing an ovarian venogram) to see if the valves are working correctly.

Treatment Options for Pelvic Congestion Syndrome

While non-steroidal anti-inflammatory drugs (NSAIDs) may help the pain of pelvic congestion syndrome, it is not a good long-term solution. The best treatment option is embolization (blockage) of the ovarian veins by an interventional radiologist. Blocking the abnormal veins keeps the blood from pooling in the pelvis. It resolves the pain and other symptoms of pelvic congestion syndrome in up to 85% of women.[44] The only other treatment option is hysterectomy with removal of the ovaries.

Other Causes of Difficult Periods

Abnormal Ovulation

If none of the problems we've already covered (fibroids, polyps, endometriosis, and adenomyosis) are the cause of abnormal uterine bleeding (AUB), it is usually due to lack of ovulation (when the ovary releases an egg) or inconsistent ovulation. Lack of ovulation can be a sign of other disorders. Premenstrual symptoms or the feeling of an impending period are absent when an egg is not produced.

When a woman first starts having periods, the organs in the brain that trigger hormone production (the pituitary and hypothalamus) are immature. This results in the lack of an egg release (no ovulation). No egg release means the ovaries cannot make enough hormones to produce a normal lining of the uterus. The abnormal lining sheds at irregular times and can be light or heavy.

Extreme exercise and weight loss, pituitary tumors, the absence of ovaries, radiation or chemotherapy can also be the reasons for lack of ovulation. Other hormonal conditions such as excess or inadequate thyroid hormone production or excess prolactin (the hormone that stimulates breast milk) from the pituitary can also interfere with ovulation.

Tests to Diagnose the Cause of Lack of Ovulation

This is a list of the laboratory tests that can be performed to help determine the cause of AUB. They are listed in order of how commonly they are required.

- Pregnancy test (HCG)

- Complete blood count (CBC)

- Thyroid function tests

- Prolactin level

- Menstrual hormone tests (FSH, LH, estradiol)

- Tests for abnormal blood clotting

- Testosterone test

- Tests for adrenal diseases

- Liver function tests

- Kidney function tests

- Tests for autoimmune diseases

- Genetic tests

Usually an ultrasound will be the only examination needed to help diagnose the cause of lack of ovulation.

Usually an ultrasound will be the only examination needed to help diagnose the cause of lack of ovulation. It allows evaluation of the ovaries for cysts or tumors. It is also very helpful for evaluation and measurement of the uterine lining. Other imaging exams that are occasionally used include an ultrasound of the thyroid gland, a CT scan to evaluate the adrenal glands, and magnetic resonance imaging (MRI) to look at the pituitary gland.

Treatment of AUB due to lack of ovulation depends on the underlying cause. Persistent ovulation problems can usually be managed with oral contraceptives, progesterone, a progesterone-containing IUD, or agents to cause ovulation if the woman wants to get pregnant. Guidelines have been developed for the treatment of abnormal uterine bleeding caused by ovulatory dysfunction from any cause.[45]

Estrogens, progestins, nonsteroidal anti-inflammatory drugs (NSAIDs), antifibrinolytics (medicines to block the breakdown of blood clots), and gonadotropin-releasing hormone analogues (GnRH) are the most commonly used agents for AUB. A reduction in blood loss has also been shown in some ovulatory patients by taking drugs that cause the blood to thicken and clot off especially when bleeding disorders are present.

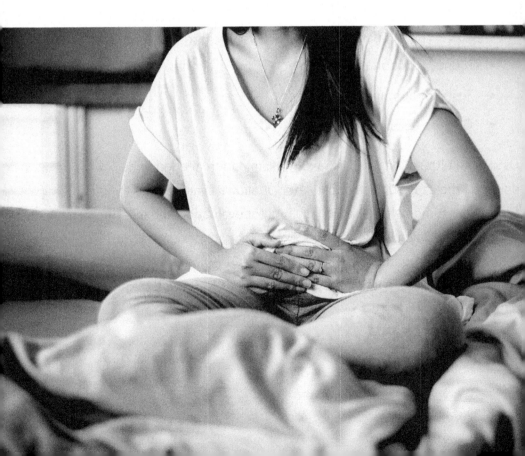

Medications

There are multiple types of medications that can cause AUB. Natural products that can do so include soy protein (in large quantities), gingko, and ginseng. Pharmaceutical medications that can cause AUB include blood thinners, aspirin, birth control pills, estrogen replacement therapy, and other types of steroids. Several medications given for psychiatric illnesses can also lead to AUB.

Polycystic Ovarian Syndrome

Polycystic ovarian syndrome (PCOS) is a well-known cause for lack of ovulation and is due to a genetic defect. The genetic defect results in multiple small cysts on the ovaries that make excess hormones such as estrogen, progesterone, and testosterone. The result is an imbalance that makes the lining shed unpredictably or not at all. Other symptoms include hair growth in unwanted places, acne, obesity, and insulin resistance.

PCOS is treated with medications such as oral contraceptives to lower testosterone levels. The insulin resistance is often treated with metformin, an oral insulin-like drug. Surgery is rarely performed except in some cases where partial removal of the ovaries can help with fertility issues from PCOS.

Bleeding Disorders

Up to 36% of women with AUB have some type of bleeding disorder. The most common one is von Willebrand disease, which is a clotting abnormality due to deficient levels of one of the clotting factors, factor 7.[46] An underlying bleeding disorder should be suspected if a woman has excessive bleeding from the time she first starts having periods or a family history of bleeding disorders. Other clues to a bleeding disorder include bruising without a known injury, bleeding gums, bleeding from the gastrointestinal tract, or nosebleeds that cannot be stopped easily.

There are medicines such as desmopressin acetate (DDAVP) that can be given to help the excessive bleeding from bleeding disorders.

Cancers

Cervical Cancer

Cervical cancer is caused by an infection with the human papilloma virus in the majority of cases. Early stages or pre-cancerous stages rarely result in bleeding and can be easily treated with outpatient minor surgical procedures. Advanced cervical cancer can cause bleeding that can sometimes be profuse. Medical management is not used in these cases. Vaginal packing, radiation, interventional radiology techniques to clog the artery supplying the tumor, and surgery in the form of hysterectomy are the primary tools to manage this type of bleeding.

> For endometrial cancer, excess estrogen exposure is the primary culprit. The excess estrogen can be due to obesity, long term lack of ovulation, or other underlying medical conditions.

Endometrial or Uterine Cancer

Uterine cancer can arise from the lining of the uterus or in other layers such as the muscle. For endometrial cancer, excess estrogen exposure is the primary culprit. The excess estrogen can be due to obesity, long term lack of ovulation, or other underlying medical conditions.

When irregular or excessive bleeding is encountered in a postmenopausal woman, an ultrasound is done to look for fibroids or other causes of AUB. If the endometrial lining is thickened, an endometrial biopsy or a D&C is performed to check for cancerous or pre-cancerous cells. If the biopsy or results of the D&C show no cancer, the woman is treated for overgrowth of the endometrium. The mainstay of this type of treatment is a progestational medicine such as norethindrone or megestrol.

If any cancerous cells are present, the treatment is hysterectomy. Postoperative radiation or chemotherapy may also be required. Premenopausal women can develop uterine cancer especially when lack of ovulation occurs long term.

Leiomyosarcoma is a muscular tumor of the uterus that arise from a muscle in the uterus. The vast majority of fibroids are benign but any rapid growth, unusual symptoms, or change in bleeding patterns should alert a woman to see her gynecologist. A leiomyosarcoma is surgically treated with a hysterectomy.

Ovarian Cancer

There are a couple of types of ovarian cancer that can cause AUB. The most common type is a granulosa cell tumor because it makes extra estrogen that makes the uterine lining grow. It can be removed surgically by removing the affected ovary or with both a hysterectomy and removal of one or both ovaries.

While there are many non-cancerous causes of miserable periods, make sure that your gynecologist rules cancer out and explains to you why he or she believes so.

Conclusion

IT'S TIME TO TAKE YOUR LIFE BACK

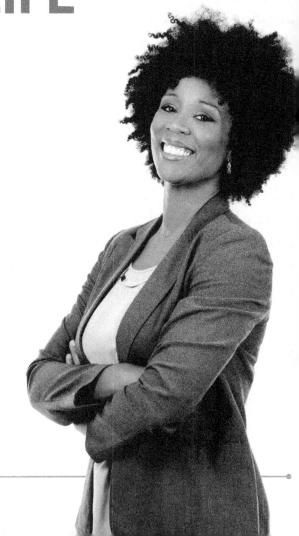

I'm a big fan of modern medicine, and especially of all the advances there have been in obstetrics, gynecology, and radiology in the last decade or two. The state of the science and technology has advanced greatly, and my aim with this book has been to introduce you to the truly amazing array of options there are for treating difficult periods. I hope that by reading the information here, you will feel empowered to take control of your uterine health once and for all. In this day and age, there is so much that can be done to alleviate your misery. You don't need to suffer like your mama and grandma did. So, untether yourself from that box of pads and drop that hot water bottle. Start exploring your options so you can start living your life again!

Even if you are like Jasmine, who I introduced at the beginning of this book, and you have become a virtual prisoner to your periods every month, know that a hysterectomy is not necessarily your only option. Although some patients in some circumstances may opt to have a hysterectomy, for most of us, losing an organ is a frightening prospect. It also may not be necessary. Therefore, arm yourself with the facts and find out which treatment option is best for you.

To help you along on your journey, I have included a flow chart below that you can use as a roadmap. I wish you more comfort, more happiness, and the best of health in the years ahead.

EVALUATION OF DIFFICULT PERIODS

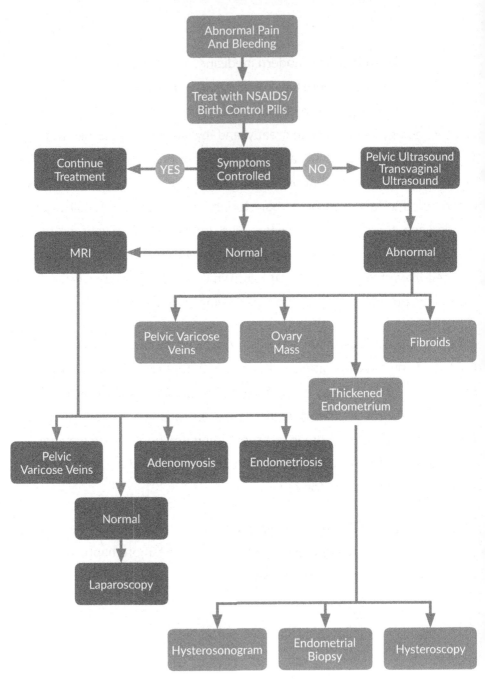

ENDNOTES

1   Liu Z, Doan QV, Blumenthal P, Dubois RW. A systematic review evaluating health-related quality of life, work impairment, and health-care costs and utilization in abnormal uterine bleeding. *Value Health* 2007 May-Jun;10(3):183-94.

2   Baird DD, Dunson DB, Hill MC, Cousins D, Schectman JM. High cumulative incidence of uterine leiomyoma in black and white women: ultrasound evidence. *Am J Obstet Gynecol.* 2003 Jan;188(1):100-7.

3   Styer AK, Rueda BR. The Epidemiology and Genetics of Uterine Leiomyoma. *Best Pract Res Clin Obstet Gynaecol.* 2016 Jul;34:3-12.

4   Moshesh M, Olshan AF, Saldana T, Baird D. Examining the relationship between uterine fibroids and dyspareunia among premenopausal women in the United States. *J Sex Med.* 2014 Mar;11(3):800-8.

5   Sundermann AC, Velez Edwards DR, Bray MJ, Jones SH, Latham SM, Hartmann KE. Leiomyomas in Pregnancy and Spontaneous Abortion: A Systematic Review and Meta-analysis. *Obstet Gynecol.* 2017 Nov;130(5):1065-1072.

6   Practice Committee of the American Society for Reproductive Medicine. Removal of myomas in asymptomatic patients to improve fertility and/or reduce miscarriage rate: a guideline. *Fertil Steril.* 2017 Sep;108(3):416-425.

7   Liu JP, Yang H, Xia Y, Cardini F. Herbal preparations for uterine fibroids. *Cochrane Database Syst Rev.* 2013 Apr 30;(4):CD005292.

8   Stenchever MA. Risks of oral contraceptive use in women over 35. *J Reprod Med.* 1993 Dec;38(12 Suppl):1030-5.

9   Leminen H, Hurskainen R. Tranexamic acid for the treatment of heavy menstrual bleeding: efficacy and safety. *Int J Women's Health.* 2012;4:413-21.

10 Kalampokas T, Kamath M, Boutas I, Kalampokas E. Ulipristal acetate for uterine fibroids: a systematic review and meta-analysis. *Gynecol Endocrinol.* 2016;32(2):91-6.

11 Munro MG. Endometrial ablation. *Best Pract Res Clin Obstet Gynaecol.* 2018 Jan;46:120-139.

12 Vashisht, A, Studd, J, Carey, A, and Burn, P. Fatal septicaemia after fibroid embolisation. *Lancet.* 1999; 354: 307–308.

13 de Blok, S, de Vries, C, Prinssen, HM, Blaauwgeers, HL, and Jorna-Meijer, LB. Fatal sepsis after uterine artery embolization with microspheres. *J Vasc Interv. Radiol.* 2003; 14: 779–783.

14 Walker WJ, McDowell SJ. Pregnancy after uterine artery embolization for leiomyomata: a series of 56 completed pregnancies. *Am J Obstet Gynecol.* 2006 Nov;195(5):1266-71.

15 Pron G, Mocarski E, Bennett J, Vilos G, Common A, Vanderburgh L; Ontario UFE Collaborative Group. Pregnancy after uterine artery embolization for leiomyomata: the Ontario multicenter trial. *Obstet Gynecol.* 2005 Jan;105(1):67-76.

16 Goldberg J, Pereira L, Berghella V, Diamond J, Daraï E, Seinera P, Seracchioli R. Pregnancy outcomes after treatment for fibromyomata: uterine artery embolization versus laparoscopic myomectomy. *Am J Obstet Gynecol.* 2004 Jul;191(1):18-21.

17 Goldberg J, Pereira L. Pregnancy outcomes following treatment for fibroids: uterine fibroid embolization versus laparoscopic myomectomy. *Curr Opin Obstet Gynecol.* 2006 Aug;18(4):402-6.

18 Pisco JM, Duarte M, Bilhim T, Branco J, Cirurgião F, Forjaz M, Fernandes L, Pereira J, Costa N, Pisco JBM, Oliveira AG. Spontaneous Pregnancy with a Live Birth after Conventional and Partial Uterine Fibroid Embolization. *Radiology.* 2017 Oct;285(1):302-310.

19 Radosa MP, Owsianowski Z, Mothes A, Weisheit A, Vorwergk J, Asskaryar FA, Camara O, Bernardi TS, Runnebaum IB. Long-term risk of fibroid recurrence after laparoscopic myomectomy. *Eur J Obstet Gynecol Reprod Biol.* 2014 Sep;180:35-9.

20 Advincula AP, Song A, Burke W, Reynolds RK. Preliminary Experience with Robot-Assisted Laparoscopic Myomectomy. *J Am Assoc Gynecol Laparosc.* 2004 Nov;11(4):511-8.

21 Jin C, Hu Y, Chen XC, Zheng FY, Lin F, Zhou K, Chen FD, Gu HZ. Laparoscopic versus open myomectomy – a meta-analysis of randomized controlled trials. *Eur J Obstet Gynecol Reprod Biol.* 2009;145(1):14–21.

22 Iavazzo C, Mamais I, Gkegkes ID. Robotic assisted vs laparoscopic and/or open myomectomy: systematic review and meta-analysis of the clinical evidence. *Arch Gynecol Obstet.* 2016 Jul;294(1):5-17.

23 United States Health and Human Services Food and Drug Administration. Laparoscopic Power Morcellators. Retrieved on February 16, 2018 from: https://www.fda.gov/medicaldevices/productsandmedicalprocedures/ surgeryandlifesupport/ucm584463.htm.

24 Radosa MP, Owsianowski Z, Mothes A, Weisheit A, Vorwergk J, Asskaryar FA, Camara O, Bernardi TS, Runnebaum IB. Long-term risk of fibroid recurrence after laparoscopic myomectomy. *Eur J Obstet Gynecol Reprod Biol.* 2014 Sep;180:35-9.

25 Katherine A. O'Hanlan, MD, Suzanne L. Dibble, DNSc, RN, Anne-Caroline Garnier, BS, andMirjam Leuchtenberger Reuland, MD. Total Laparoscopic Hysterectomy: Technique and Complications of 830 Cases. *JSLS.* 2007 Jan-Mar; 11(1): 45–53.

26 Martino MA, Berger EA, McFetridge JT, Shubella J, Gosciniak G, Wejkszner T, Kainz GF, Patriarco J, Thomas MB, Boulay R. A comparison of quality outcome measures in patients having a hysterectomy for benign disease: robotic vs. non-robotic approaches. *J Minim Invasive Gynecol.* 2014 May-Jun;21(3):389-93.

27 Laughlin-Tommaso SK, Khan Z, Weaver AL, Smith CY, Rocca WA, Stewart EA. Cardiovascular and metabolic morbidity after hysterectomy with ovarian conservation: a cohort study. *Menopause.* 2018 May;25(5):483-492.

28 Dreisler E, Stampe Sorensen S, Ibsen PH, Lose G. Prevalence of endometrial polyps and abnormal uterine bleeding in a Danish population aged 20-74 years. *Ultrasound Obstet Gynecol.* 2009 Jan;33(1):102-8.

29 Sasaki LMP, Andrade KRC, Figueiredo ACMG, Wanderley MDS, Pereira MG. Factors Associated with Malignancy in Hysteroscopically Resected Endometrial Polyps: A Systematic Review and Meta-Analysis. *J Minim Invasive Gynecol*. 2018 Feb 14.

30 Lee SC, Kaunitz AM, Sanchez-Ramos L, Rhatigan RM. The oncogenic potential of endometrial polyps: a systematic review and meta-analysis. *Obstet Gynecol*. 2010 Nov;116(5):1197-205.

31 Lobo RA. Endometriosis: etiology, pathology, diagnosis, management. *Comprehensive Gynecology*. Philadelphia, PA: Mosby; 5th ed. 2007:chap 19.

32 Zullo F, Spagnolo E, Saccone G, Acunzo M, Xodo S, Ceccaroni M, Berghella V. Endometriosis and obstetrics complications: a systematic review and meta-analysis. *Fertil Steril*. 2017 Oct;108(4):667-672.e5.

33 Wheeler JM. Epidemiology of endometriosis-associated infertility. *J Reprod Med*. 1989 Jan. 34(1):41-6.

34 Buchweitz O, Poel T, Diedrich K, Malik E. The diagnostic dilemma of minimal and mild endometriosis under routine conditions. *J Am Assoc Gynecol Laparosc*. 2003 Feb. 10(1):85-9.

35 Flower A, Liu JP, Lewith G, Little P, Li Q. Chinese herbal medicine for endometriosis. *Cochrane Database of Systematic Reviews* 2012, Issue 5. Art. No.: CD006568.

36 Kauppila A. Changing concepts of medical treatment of endometriosis. *Acta Obstet Gynecol Scand*. 1993 Jul. 72(5):324-36.

37 Schlaff WD, Dugoff L, Damewood MD, Rock JA. Megestrol acetate for treatment of endometriosis. *Obstet Gynecol*. 1990 Apr. 75(4):646-8.

38 Sutton CJ, Pooley AS, Ewen SP, Haines P. Follow-up report on a randomized controlled trial of laser laparoscopy in the treatment of pelvic pain associated with minimal to moderate endometriosis. *Fertil Steril*. 1997 Dec. 68(6):1070-4.

39 Waller KG, Shaw RW. Gonadotropin-releasing hormone analogues for the treatment of endometriosis: long-term follow-up. *Fertil Steril*. 1993 Mar. 59(3):511-5.

40 Leyendecker G, Wildt L, Mall G. The pathophysiology of endometriosis and adenomyosis: tissue injury and repair. *Arch Gynecol Obstet*. 2009 Oct. 280 (4):529-38.

41 Taran FA, Stewart EA, Brucker S. Adenomyosis: Epidemiology, Risk Factors, Clinical Phenotype and Surgical and Interventional Alternatives to Hysterectomy. *Geburtshilfe Frauenheilkd.* 2013 Sep. 73 (9):924-931.

42 Mayo JL. A healthy menstrual cycle. *Clinical Nutrition Insights* 1997, 5(9):1-8.

43 de Bruijn AM, Smink M, Lohle PNM, Huirne JAF, Twisk JWR, Wong C, Schoonmade L, Hehenkamp WJK.Uterine artery embolization for the treatment of adenomyosis: A systematic review and meta-analysis. *J Vasc Interv Radiol.* 2017 Dec;28(12):1629-1642.

44 Kim HS, Malhotra AD, Rowe PC, et al. Embolotherapy for pelvic congestion syndrome: long-term results. *J Vasc Interv Radiol.* 2006;17(2 Pt 1):289-297.

45 Committee on Practice Bulletins—Gynecology. Practice bulletin no. 136: Management of abnormal uterine bleeding associated with ovulatory dysfunction. *Obstet Gynecol.* 2013 Jul. 122 (1):176-85.

46 Deligeorglou E, Karountzos V. Abnormal Uterine Bleeding including coagulopathies and other menstrual disorders. *Best Pract Res Clin Obstet Gynaecol.* 2018 Apr;48:51-61.

Made in the USA
Las Vegas, NV
14 September 2022

55302400R00083